new
lives

new
lives

Nurses' Stories
about Caring
for Babies

Kathleen Huggins, RN, MS Editor

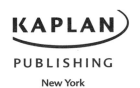

PUBLISHING

New York

This publication is designed to provide accurate and authoritative information in regard to the subject matter covered. It is sold with the understanding that the publisher is not engaged in rendering medical, legal, or other professional service. If legal advice or other expert assistance is required, the services of a competent professional should be sought.

Published by Kaplan Publishing, a division of Kaplan, Inc.

1 Liberty Plaza, 24th Floor

New York, NY 10006

While the stories in this anthology are based on real events, names, places, and other details have been changed for the sake of privacy.

Printed in the United States of America

10 9 8 7 6 5 4 3 2 1

Library of Congress Cataloging-in-Publication Data
New lives: nurses' stories about caring for babies/[edited by] Kathleen Huggins.
    p.; cm. — (Kaplan voices)
  ISBN 978-1-4277-9965-4
  1. Newborn infants—Diseases—Nursing. I. Huggins, Kathleen.
II. Series: Kaplan voices.
  [DNLM: 1. Neonatal Nursing—Personal Narratives. 2. Nurses—psychology—Personal Narratives. WY 157.3 N532 2009]
  RJ245.N487 2009
  618.92'01–dc22

                        2008055652

Kaplan Publishing books are available at special quantity discounts to use for sales promotions, employee premiums, or educational purposes. Please email our Special Sales Department to order or for more information at kaplanpublishing@kaplan.com, or write to Kaplan Publishing, 1 Liberty Plaza, 24th Floor, New York, NY 10006.

Contents

Introduction ix

PART ONE: Neophyte Learning 1

Amy, the Ad, and Adam 3
Carole Kenner, DNS, RNC-NIC, FAAN

A Gut Feeling 9
Dianna M. Hannah, RN

The Baby in the Ambulance 21
Bonnie Jarvis-Lowe, RN

PART TWO: When Birth Ends in Sorrow 27

A Sad but True Story I Will Never Forget 29
Robin A. Roots, RN, IBCLC

Memoirs from an "Angel of Mercy" 35
Heather Tempest, RN, PNC(c)

PART THREE: Supporting Parents 41

When a Baby's Short Life Is at Home 43
Cara Bicking, RNC, BSN

Circle of Life 49
Kelly Maidment, RN

Better Late Than Never. 57
Dawn M. Kersula, MA, RN, FACCE, IBCLC

Ayub: A Parent's Story of Fear, Love, and
Determination. 61
Suzanna M. Feliciano, BSN, RN, CCRN

PART FOUR: When Nurses Bond 69

Baby Jamie, Who I Promise Not to Forget 71
Carol Blair-Murdoch, RN, BSCN

David's Miracle 77
Lanette L. Anderson, MSN, JD, RN

PART FIVE: Lessons Learned 83

Stolen Time 85
Margie Marier-Porchia, RN, BS

In God's Palm 91
Nancy Leigh Harless, ARNP

A New Life in My Charge. 99
Karen Klein, RN

My Story 107
Monica Frommer, RN

Changing Assignments 111
Nicole M. Jarrell, MSN, RNC

Icarus Again. 121
Julianna Paradisi, RN

The Cath Lab Baby 131
  Vera Knox, RNC

PART SIX: Nurses Who Challenge 141

Emily 143
  Patricia Harman, RN, CNM, MSN

Voyagers 155
  Julianna Paradisi, RN

The Inseparable Unit 161
  Barbara Latterner, BSN, RN, IBCLC

Acknowledgment of Permissions 169

Reader's Guide 171

About the Editor 177

About the Contributors 179

Labor of Love–Preview 187

Introduction

FEW AREAS OF nursing have grown as rapidly or are as complex as perinatal nursing. Only 35 years ago, when I was beginning my career, maternity nurses were just beginning to learn about equipment for fetal monitoring and understand how to interpret fetal heart rate patterns. Ultrasound evaluations and amniocentesis were unheard of. Few nurse midwives practiced in American hospitals.

Mothers birthed alone without the support of loved ones. Many were so sedated during birth, they had little memory of the delivery of their child. Tiny premature babies were placed in warmed isolettes and prayed for. Oxygen was pumped into the baby's bed with little understanding of the risk of blindness.

Not that long ago, fetal and newborn deaths were shielded from parents due to the mistaken belief that this would help them suffer less over their loss. Mothers primarily fed formula to their newborns, and in 1971, breast-feeding rates were at an all-time low. Doctors actively discouraged women from breastfeeding and the use of the "dry up" shot was commonplace. There was no such profession as lactation consultant.

But over the past few decades, the specialties of obstetrical nursing, neonatal care, and lactation has exploded. A new graduate or nurse transferring into these fields has much to learn before she or he is ready to care for mothers and infants in his or her charge.

Many, including the public at large, neophytes, and nurses in other specialties, may envision the obstetrical and newborn professions as a work environment filled with joy and satisfaction as babies come into the world. While nurses who work with newborns certainly do enjoy fulfillment in their chosen field, they also experience pressure and anxiety from challenging situations and frustration from both physicians and co-workers, as well as disappointment and sorrow.

The 20 stories included in this anthology represent a broad range of nursing perspectives from nurses who work in a variety of the subspecialties of perinatal nursing. The growing technology in neonatology is evident and one can only begin to appreciate how overwhelmed new parents of sick newborns must be and what a job it is for nurses to help families bond with their critically ill infants. The writers reveal both the joy and disappointment from the delivery room.

The stories expose a multitude of situations in which both novices and seasoned professionals learn valuable lessons while caring for newborns and their families, including helping them grieve over their losses. Included are stories of nurses' heroic efforts in situations where they are inexperienced and frightened. The stories make clear that infants and parents who come into a nurse's care leave an indelible imprint in their memories.

new
lives

PART ONE

Neophyte Learning

Amy, the Ad, and Adam

~

Carole Kenner, DNS, RNC-NIC, FAAN

CIRCUMSTANCES AND PEOPLE are often like books and movies; some make a lasting impression while others are quickly forgotten. Likewise, unforgettable and indelible experiences are interposed within a framework of education and empirical evidence, eventually giving rise to a nurse's professional philosophy. As a young nurse in the neonatal intensive care unit, I was dedicated to learning as much as I could to provide the specialized care necessary to assist premature babies in overcoming the odds. Looking back, I realize that in my quest to master the clinical complexities of an intensive care setting, I was still on a learning curve when integrating the holistic and psychological/social aspects of nursing care. Granted, technical expertise plays a critical role in patient outcomes and should never be underestimated.

But even the best nurses may compartmentalize their jobs into a series of skilled interventions performed in an eight-to-twelve-hour shift.

Early in my career, the seeds were planted for the focus of my doctoral research: parent transition from the NICU back into the community and the home. Although a number of factors had broadened my outlook and contributed to a more inclusive stance when testing models of care delivery and examining patient outcomes, one young mother and her child played a pivotal role in my professional development and ultimately, in my body of research.

Quite simply, Amy and Adam taught me valuable lessons that are easy to overlook in the hustle and bustle of a high-tech NICU environment: providing quality nursing care for infants and children must be delivered within the context of the family unit, and caution must always be exercised before making assumptions about a patient or a family's level of knowledge.

At 14, Amy was a child who gave birth to a child. Although unwed teen pregnancy was becoming more common in the 1970s, Amy had been disowned by her parents and the baby's father was nowhere in sight. Waiflike and vulnerable, the young mother had no choice but to walk this path alone.

Like most mothers, Amy wanted her baby to be healthy, with a future filled with hope and opportunity. However, Adam was born extremely premature, and his prognosis was grim from the outset.

As Amy began to open up, we learned that in addition to coping with her son's physical condition and the many foreign and frightening experiences that accompany care in a NICU, she was dealing with guilt. In her heart of hearts, Amy knew she was too young to be a mother, and yet she'd given birth to a severely premature baby when she was unprepared to take care of him. And while she was afraid and at times overwhelmed, she also possessed an inner strength in the face of adversity that many new mothers—regardless of age—may lack.

At the time, palliative care was in its infancy, and neonatal professionals were early proponents of the provision of comfort and solace when wellness isn't an option. As Adam deteriorated, we prepared Amy for the inevitable, assuring the young mother that her baby's suffering would be minimal.

In Adam's final hours, we disconnected all IVs and monitor leads, allowing Amy to hold her son without encumbrances. As new mothers are wont to do, she ran her fingers through his wispy brown hair and kissed his forehead. As if to reaffirm that which was normal about her son, she examined his small fingers and toes, one by one. Swaddling him once more, she held him to her chest and gently began to rock.

Watching this ancient mother/child ritual, I knew that even though Adam was beyond intervention, his mother was in need of nursing care. I sat beside her quietly.

After a moment, she turned and asked, "How much does that ad cost?"

I was confused. "What ad?"

"When someone dies, they put an ad in the paper," she said. "Do you know how much it costs?"

Amy was referring to an obituary, a scenario that hadn't been covered in nursing school. Before I could respond, she added, "There's something else I've been thinking about. What will happen to Adam after he dies? I don't have the money to bury him. Will they just throw him in the trash?"

Few questions have carried such enormous impact. I was proficient at interpreting blood gases and acid-base balance. I understood the etiology of hyperbilirubenemia, its signs and symptoms, treatment modalities, and long-term complications. I could visually assess a neonate's respiratory pattern rapidly, identifying signs of stress and impending respiratory failure in order to intervene proactively. But I realized I could not easily answer her questions. I really did not have enough life experiences myself to be sure how to guide her.

I didn't know how to place an obituary in the local newspaper. And while I was aware that the city had a pauper's cemetery, I didn't know the procedure involved in making burial arrangements. However, I did know our hospital's staff included an interdisciplinary team of professionals who were available to meet the diverse needs of our patients and their families.

"I'll call the chaplain and a social worker," I said. "We'll find answers to your questions together."

And we did. Many years later, I hope I made a difference in Amy's life by listening and offering assistance and support during a traumatic and difficult time. I do know she made a difference in mine. Amy and Adam taught me that if I didn't take care of the family, I didn't take care of the baby. Building on this principle and extending it beyond the walls of the hospital, I focused my doctoral research on improving neonatal outcomes by identifying problem areas common to all parents, regardless of cultural or socioeconomic differences. An integral part of my study included making home visits to assess the family unit post-discharge, providing a bridge from the highly technical but structured and protected environment in a NICU to the day-to-day realities awaiting parents as they face a world of unknowns.

When making home visits in rural America, I've chased cows out of the road. In foreign countries, I've hiked mountainous trails to huts with dirt floors that house multiple human generations, as well as flocks of chickens and roosters. The methodology and tools developed from my research have provided the basis for NICU discharge planning protocols in the United States, and the study has been replicated in many national and international sites.

The journey from Amy and Adam until the present has borne much fruit, including my desire to advocate for the health of infants and children around the world. In

2005, I founded the Council of International Neonatal Nurses, or COINN. The acronym is synonymous with the value children have to our future.

Perhaps on a small scale, technological advances that now save the tiniest of babies—some weighing under a pound and as early as 22 to 23 weeks' gestation—are somewhat analogous to America's space program. Quoting Neil Armstrong, another Ohioan, as he walked on the moon, it might be said that the NICU represents "one small step for man." However, raising the standard of care for neonates and children across the globe represents "one giant leap for mankind."

A Gut Feeling

~

Dianna M. Hannah, RN

It was an average Saturday morning in early January. I got to work just on time as usual. I sat in report and listened to the night-shift charge nurse give a brief overall report of the patients. Nothing out of the ordinary. I remember thinking it was going to be an average, typical, ordinary day on Mother/Baby . . . or was it? Little did I realize that it would be a day I'd never forget as long as I lived.

I had been on Mother/Baby for only about six months. Before that I worked on a Medical/Surgical floor for one and a half years and before that, at a northern Virginia hospital's emergency department for seven months as a new graduate nurse. Although I had little experience with adult patients and even less with newborn babies, I felt comfortable on the postpartum floor. Not only were the patients usually stable, but I was also surrounded by a great staff of experienced nurses. Many of the nurses had been there 20 to 30 years or more.

I had been given a typical assignment of four moms and four babies. I got report from the night-shift nurses, checked my charts, reviewed medication times, and prioritized my care accordingly. I remember beginning my care with a new mother of a 35-week infant that was born by cesarean section. I don't remember why he was born so early. I think she went into preterm labor, or maybe it was pregnancy-induced hypertension. I did know that she'd had a late miscarriage prior to conceiving him, and both she and her husband were very nervous about this child. I remembered in report that the baby, whom I'll call Sam Doe, spent approximately 12 hours in the neonatal intensive care unit, or NICU, just after birth because of unexplained low oxygen saturations. After his O$_2$ sats were within normal range and he appeared to be doing fine, he was transferred to the floor with his parents.

I knocked on the door as I glanced down at my report sheet. Someone from inside softly said, "Come in." I opened the door and went inside.

Smiling, I said, "Good morning. My name is Dianna and I will be your nurse today until about three o'clock." The lights were dim in the room, but I could see the mother nursing her baby in bed and a larger person sleeping soundly on the couch on the far side of the room. I assessed how well the baby was latched and sucking, as well as how comfortable the mother was with nursing him. Sam was a little over five pounds. He looked tiny in his mother's arms, but he was breastfeeding well. As I stood beside the bed talking to her, he released his latch and began to fall asleep. I asked her if I could examine him. She said yes, so I picked him up and placed him in his crib. I remember distinctly at that moment looking at him and feeling as though I was looking at a dead baby. I could see his chest rise and fall so I knew he was breathing, but his color was very disturbing. His skin was a shade of pale yellow that I had never seen before. I asked Sam's mother if I could turn on the brighter room light so I could see him better.

"Sure," she said. "Is something wrong?" I imagine she could see the concern in my eyes, although I tried to hide it.

"I just want to see him under better lighting. The lights in these rooms are so bad," I answered. I checked his vital signs and listened carefully to his lungs. Everything was within normal range.

She again asked me, "Is he okay?"

"He's fine," I answered, but my gut feeling told me otherwise. With my little experience and this mother's nervousness, I felt that I'd be jumping the gun and might cause unnecessary worry if I took the baby immediately to the nursery to examine him. But I also felt there were several experienced nurses there that could quickly put my worries to rest.

As a new nurse I doubted myself many times. I remember thinking that I was probably worried for nothing. The baby's vital signs were within normal limits, he was nursing well, and I knew the pediatrician would be in shortly. I wrote everything down on his flow sheet and washed my hands. I began writing my name and cell phone number on her wipe-off board when my phone rang.

"Please bring baby Doe to the nursery. Dr. Purks is on her way to see him," the nursery nurse said.

"Okay," I said. A feeling of relief came over me. I explained to Sam's mother and waking father that the doctor was on her way and I needed to take Sam to the nursery. I showed them the yellow passport card and wheeled the crib out.

When I arrived at the nursery, I asked the nursery nurse to look at the baby. She had 25 to 30 years of experience, so I trusted her opinion. She examined him and said, "What do you think is wrong?"

"Does his color look funny to you?" I asked.

"Well," she answered, "he *is* a little pale and a little yellow. But not out of the ordinary for a 35-weeker." I knew it. I was worried for nothing. I lay the infant back in his crib and left the nursery to finish checking other patients.

A while later I returned to the nursery to check Sam's chart for new orders. I noticed Dr. Purks had seen him. She'd written for a complete blood count, or CBC, and bilirubin STAT. I read her progress notes, which mainly stated the baby looked pale and slightly jaundiced. I put the chart back on the desk and drew the secretary's attention to it. I took another look at Sam before I began to assess an infant whose crib was next to his. Strangely, I felt the same thing I'd felt earlier. I still sensed that something was terribly wrong with him. Why was I feeling like that?

I called another Mother/Baby nurse over to look at him. "Does he look okay to you?" I asked her. She looked him over and said, "Umm…he looks okay. Why?" "I don't know," I said. "I just get a weird feeling about him." However, I again doubted myself and shrugged if off, thinking that if I said anything further I'd be overreacting.

The neonatologist who'd discharged Sam from the NICU was in the nursery at that time. I asked her what she thought. She explained that she thought he was fine and that Dr. Purks had already examined him.

Okay, I said to myself. The nurse, pediatrician, and neonatologist all thought Sam was fine. I was the only one who was worried. And who was I? I was an inexperienced nurse who'd only examined babies for six months. What did I know?

I grabbed Sam's crib and headed toward the door. Looking down at him, I again got an uneasy feeling. To me, he really looked dead lying in his crib. His eyes were closed and he had such a strange color.

"Are you sure he's okay?" I asked the nursery nurse again. I'm sure I was getting on her nerves, but she stopped what she was doing and examined him with me again. We noticed his nostrils flare a couple of times. When babies have flaring nostrils, it can be a sign of respiratory distress. Sam, however, only had occasional flaring and no other problems.

"Look . . . Dianna," she said, "if you are really that worried, put him on the pulse ox monitor." I agreed that would put my worries to rest. I placed it on his foot and turned on the monitor. It immediately went up to 95 percent.

"Ninety-five isn't bad," she said. Agreeing with her, I again felt relieved. I stood by the crib for about 10 or 15 minutes longer, making sure his O_2 sats wouldn't drop. He *was* fine, I thought. However, as I turned to walk away, the alarm sounded. The monitor dropped to 90 percent and within a few minutes, down to 89 percent, then 88 percent and 87 percent. I remember someone suggesting I might have placed it on his foot wrong, or maybe he'd kicked it loose. I almost agreed until I saw how fast he was breathing. His respirations were 80 to 100 breaths per minute. I remember counting over and over again, hoping I was counting wrong.

Something *was* wrong with him. I paged Dr. Purks immediately. Within five minutes she walked through the nursery door. Not knowing yet that I'd paged her, she looked over and said, "What's going on with Mr. Doe?"

"His sats dropped and he's become tachypneic," I answered.

"I had a feeling about him," she said. "Transfer him to the NICU as soon as possible."

I immediately went to his mother's room to give her the update on Sam. I knocked on the door and went in. "Has the doctor called or been in to see you about the baby?" I asked.

"No. Not yet. Why?" she asked. "What's wrong?"

"His oxygen saturations dropped again and he's breathing faster than he should," I answered. Tears filled her tired eyes as she tried to remain strong. "Do you think he'll be all right?" she asked. "Well, he's being transferred back to the NICU," I replied. "He's going to be okay. He's in the best place he can be. They can watch him a lot more closely than we can on the floor. It's more one-on-one in the NICU." I actually believed he would be fine and would be there for just a short while for observation. I'd soon find out that I'd broken the cardinal rule of nursing. That is, no matter how badly I wanted to comfort Sam's parents and take away their pain or worries, I should never have told them that he would be okay, since I didn't know that for sure myself.

There was a knock on the door and the neonatologist entered. He began to explain to Mr. and Mrs. Doe all the tests that would be done as I left the room. I remember feeling somewhat relieved at that moment that Sam was in the NICU, but at the same time, my heart went out to his parents.

No longer consumed with thoughts of Sam's condition, I moved on to see other patients. About 20 minutes after I'd left the Does' room, my phone rang. It was the neonatologist. "I want Mom and Dad in the room NOW," he urged, referring to the Does. I was really scared. What was going on? My first thought was that he'd coded. He hadn't, thank God. I quickly went to their room. I knocked once but no one answered. I opened the door and noticed the shower running. I knocked on the bathroom door. Mr. Doe was helping Mrs. Doe undress. She was not yet in the shower.

"The doctor is coming to talk to you both right now," I said. "Don't get in the shower yet."

"Okay," she said. "Do you know what's going on?"

"I don't," I replied. "But it sounded urgent."

She quickly dressed, and both she and her husband took a seat on the couch. Not a minute later, the doctor walked in the room. He gave them the terrible news that Sam had hypoplastic left heart syndrome and would need to be transferred immediately to a hospital in Richmond for open heart surgery or he would die. I remember thinking that I'd known something was wrong with him, but I never thought it would be something that serious. I left the room as the doctor continued talking. Before leaving, I asked Mr. Doe if there was anything I could get for them.

He replied, "Yeah . . . can you get us a two-day-old healthy heart?" as tears streamed down his cheeks. I felt awful. I somehow felt as though part of their pain was my fault. If only I hadn't told them that Sam would be okay. They'd trusted me, and now they probably hated me.

I went home that night, kissed my son, and did an Internet search for hypoplastic left heart syndrome. I gathered as much information as I could find. I even searched message boards to see how well other babies did that had been born with the same defect. There were many stories with poor outcomes. I was scared for Sam, but at least he had a chance.

I gathered as much information as I could find, including this description from the American Heart Association:

> In Hypoplastic Left Heart Syndrome, the left side of the heart—including the aorta, aortic valve, left ventricle and mitral valve—is under-developed. Blood returning from the lungs must flow through an opening in the wall between the atria (atrial septal defect). The right ventricle pumps the blood into the pulmonary artery and blood reaches the aorta through a patent ductus arteriosus.
>
> The baby often seems normal at birth, but will come to medical attention within a few days of birth as the ductus closes. Babies with this syndrome become ashen, have rapid and difficult breathing and have difficulty feeding. This heart defect is usually fatal within the first days or months of life unless it's treated.
>
> Although this defect is not correctable, some babies can be treated with a series of operations, or a heart transplantation. Until an operation is performed, the ductus is kept open by intravenous medication.

I returned to work the next day with a better under-standing of Sam's diagnosis but nervous about facing his parents. I heard in report that Mrs. Doe was discharged, and was a little relieved that I didn't have to face her. But after coming out of report, someone said we had no sup-port staff to push the wheelchair out, so I was asked to take Mrs. Doe down to her car. I still had to see her. I took a wheelchair to her room and knocked on the door. I was terrified to face her. I took a deep breath and opened the door.

"Hi. How are you?" I softly asked. She looked up from what she was doing and before I knew it, she ran over to me and hugged me. We both began to cry. "I'm so sorry," I said. After a minute we released our embrace.

She said, "I know you're the one. You knew some-thing wasn't right with him the minute you met us."

"Well . . . , " I replied, "I got a gut feeling I couldn't explain. I think God knew I couldn't have handled it if something had happened to Sam while he was in your room."

She smiled and handed me a bouquet of wildflowers. "These are for you," she said. "It's the least we can do."

"Thank you," I said.

She sat down in the wheelchair and I pushed her off the unit alongside her husband. It was a quiet walk down to their car, and I wondered what they must have been thinking. What a nightmare it must have felt like to be in their shoes! As we got closer to their car, I saw her mother waiting at the opened car door. I could tell that she had been crying as well.

"She's the one, Mom!" Mrs. Doe said as she pointed to me. I have to admit it made me feel uncomfortable to get that kind of attention. I smiled politely. She got out of the wheelchair and started to cry again. I hugged her, and she agreed she'd keep me informed on Sam's progress.

Mr. and Mrs. Doe updated me via e-mail on how Sam was doing. He did have the surgery one week later. They had to wait to operate, because he had developed an infection in his bloodstream that had to be treated first. During that week they gave him medicine to keep his ductus arteriosus open. A few months later he had a second surgery. It was a long, hard road for Sam and his parents, but he pulled through. Over the years I've received many updates and photos. My favorite picture was one of Sam wearing a green frog costume for Halloween. I was also invited to his first birthday party. Although extremely flattered to get an invitation, I kindly declined. I guess I was afraid of the attention I might have received. It's been two years, and I still get Christmas cards from them. One year ago they had a new addition to their family, a little sister for Sam. Sam is still looking at a third, less risky surgery in the future. I'm sure he will do great.

Today, I precept many new nurses and students and I almost always share this story. I want them to understand that no matter how inexperienced they are, they should *never* ignore a "gut feeling."

The Baby in the Ambulance

~

Bonnie Jarvis-Lowe, RN

IT WAS MY first job as a new registered nurse, working
at Grand Bank Cottage Hospital in Grand Bank, a little
place on the south coast of Newfoundland. A classmate
of mine, Shirley Best, was also working there, although
we saw very little of each other due to our shift rotations.
Also, I lived in the nurses' residence attached to the hospital itself and Shirley lived in the town. But we made
time once in awhile to have tea, compare experiences and
challenges, and catch up on our personal lives. She liked
it at the little hospital, as did I.

One of the first things I learned at that little hospital was how resourceful and practical all the nurses
were, how they could think so fast on their feet, and how
pleased they were to have extra pairs of hands to help
them. They were excellent teachers and we soon learned

the most efficient way to run a clinic, the quick assessments of trauma patients, and how to keep a good, level head in the midst of chaos. Those nurses were good, and that was the way we wanted to be: efficient and good at whatever was thrown our way.

When we applied for positions as graduation from the Grace Hospital School of Nursing approached, we were amazed at how many choices we had. They needed nurses all along the coasts of Newfoundland, but we were never sorry about our choice of Grand Bank. The hands-on experiences, the good teaching, the adventure, and the resourcefulness we learned have stayed with me always, and I hope that I passed them on to others.

Two doctors stand out vividly in my mind: Dr. Oliver, with his old-world genteel attitude, and Dr. Wrixon, with his boisterous run down the corridor and pole vault over the nurses' desk, and then his laugh at the havoc he had created. The same Dr. Wrixon went on to become a well-known obstetrician in Halifax, Nova Scotia. He was smart and young, and Dr. Oliver would give him a glance over his glasses from time to time, taming him for an hour or so. It was fun, and there was so much to learn from these men.

The nurses were served afternoon tea in the old English tradition, a leftover from Newfoundland's colonial days no doubt. Meals were cooked on night shifts for the workers, and all in all for us children of the baby boom, the 1960s were good to us. Our way of dress raised eyebrows from time to time, but as long as our work was good we were fine. Those were the days when nurses did not even pay unemployment insurance premiums, the reasoning being that there would always be jobs for nurses, something that would change radically in the years to come.

However, a rude awakening was in the wings for me, and it came—as most do—when I least expected it. I was doing laundry in the basement of the hospital on a cold, snowy evening when I heard the running of footsteps and my last name being called. That also was a tradition, the use of our last names for any- and everything. It was a senior nurse calling to me. It seems they had a very sick newborn baby suffering convulsions and he needed to go to the Janeway Children's Hospital in St. John's, four or five hours away, by ambulance, right away. I was there and available and was commissioned to go. So I ran to put a bit of order to myself and reported to the Outpatients Department. Dr. Wrixon passed me a bag of medications and syringes, gave me a quick run-down and a half dozen papers, and said to medicate whenever it was necessary and to keep oxygen on the babe at all times.

We headed out the emergency room door to the waiting ambulance, and started to load and hook up the oxygen. Dr. Wrixon was doing his last check when I heard a voice calling my name. I turned to see my classmate, Shirley, running through the snow, shouting, "I can't let you go alone on that road. I'm coming too!" She made room for herself in spite of my protests, and off we went.

The highway was icy, the visibility very poor, and the baby convulsed frequently. I cannot express how glad and relieved I was to have another nurse with me. We kept our stethoscopes on that little chest, our hands pushed through the hole of the isolette, changing places from time to time when we became cramped, and laughed at one point when Larry, our driver, said if only we were just two feet tall we wouldn't have that problem!

Then followed disaster—a flat tire, with not another vehicle on the road—and precious time was taken up while Larry, in his thin spring coat and in freezing temperature, changed it. Grave concern set in. This was a much longer trip than usual, we might run out of oxygen, our gas gauge might drop too low, and our power might give out, disabling our much-needed suction device—so many things ran through our minds. While we talked and shared our concerns, the baby finally fell into a medication-induced sleep and his seizures lessened.

After seven and a half hours we saw the lights of the city. Larry speeded up the ambulance and we flew across that snow-covered bit of civilization toward the Janeway Hospital, where a fresh-faced group of doctors and nurses just coming on duty ran out to meet us. After a report to the doctor, we crawled and dragged our cramped limbs into our ambulance and headed back to Grand Bank.

We had accomplished a difficult mission, and as two 21-year-old new nurses we were thrilled and proud. I was so grateful to Shirley, and as we stopped for gas and loaded up on junk food we shared our concerns about our trip. But it was finished, and the baby, we later discovered, did well; he is probably grown and a father of his own children now.

I learned so much that night. First of all, I learned to dress warmly, which I had not done; to take food and water, which I had not done; to get good doctor's orders and lots of the required medication, which I had been given; and when at all possible, to take a classmate along to help.

I did many ambulance trips after that, in many different places. But none would equal that miserable night of the blizzard and the sick baby. The paramedics were better trained, and the ambulances had more high-tech equipment, including heart monitors. The seats in the back of the vans were more comfortable, with more head room, and with speakers available to communicate with a driver up front. Yes, everything changed for the better, and the more calls I did, the better I got at that type of nursing. But no matter what, I learned the most on that snowy night in Newfoundland in 1969, a December night, with the next morning dawning still, the sunrise awesome, and the snow a carpet of marshmallow with twinkling crystals, as two young nurses, proud as peacocks, and our devoted driver headed back to a little hospital where everyone waited at the doorway to make sure we were okay and to feed and comfort us.

Never to be forgotten, it was a learning experience and an experience of the soul. As we sat our sore bodies down to eat lunch and tell Dr. Wrixon all about his patient, he jumped up and gave us both a huge bear hug, and we knew we were appreciated.

That and getting the news that the baby was doing well by then was one of the best moments of our lives.

PART TWO

When Birth Ends in Sorrow

A Sad but True Story I Will Never Forget

~

Robin A. Roots, RN, IBCLC

THE PATIENT'S ROOM was dark as I entered, in sharp contrast to the usual bright, bubbly excitement that accompanies a family welcoming the miracle of new life. I was regretting having taken this assignment as I walked down the hall to the last room. The room we reserved for this sort of thing. Thinking stupidly that the room was far enough away that this mom would not hear the crying of babies filling their lungs with air, new life she would not know this day. I felt a bit obligated to take this patient, because although it was my friend and staff nurse co-worker's turn, she was pregnant, and I did not want her to have to take the next fetal demise. I did not want her to go through this heart-wrenching ordeal at this time in her life. The patient in room 260 was quiet as I gently introduced myself. She had brought her mom with her for comfort and support during the tragic event she was about to endure. Hushed hellos were spoken, and not much eye contact was made.

When I tell people I am a labor and delivery nurse, they naturally assume it's great fun and exciting all of the time. Most people don't know the other side to this nursing specialty—the side only the physicians and nurses see. Even in this day and age, I have been around to support fathers grieving the loss of their wives, mostly due to a pulmonary embolism, or the heart-wrenching tragedy of a term stillbirth. Sometimes, despite all our modern technology, during the peripartum period events go terribly wrong and families expecting to take home the "perfect" baby do not. No one really wants to hear about babies being stillborn or even let that into their imagination. I can't blame people; I don't either. I don't like to think about the times when I am rushing a patient down the hall for a crash cesarean section, or when a cord falls out of the vagina ahead of the baby, necessitating a truly life-threatening emergency for the fetus.

It is hard to wrap your head around a husband and wife filled with excitement, counting contractions all the way to the hospital, only to have their hearts torn out, their lives and future suddenly snatched away. Expectant grandparents await the arrival of the beloved baby. No, nobody but the nurses, patients, and physicians see how such a happy time of life can turn on a dime to be the most life-shattering time instead.

My patient had come all the way from the Philippines to deliver her baby. She was a highly respected attorney in her homeland, where in some areas it is unusual for women to be in such highly successful and respected jobs. Only her closest family and friends knew about the pregnancy, but she was too far along with child now to hide her heavy belly. She had been seen at the expected intervals by her obstetrician, and all was going well until she went in for a routine checkup at 38 weeks. I can't imagine the shock and dread as the physician casually put the Doppler to her swollen belly to hear the familiar beats like a horse's hoofs . . . and heard nothing. The physician probably said something like "it must be my machine" and sent her to the hospital for an ultrasound. The patient herself must have known. Missing the familiar kicks that came like clockwork, she'd told herself the baby must be sleeping.

Ultrasound confirmed what both patient and doctor already knew. Now she was here for an induction. It was too risky for the mom to go through the stress of a C-section when the outcome for the unborn was already known. It strikes me as almost cruel to make these moms go through labor and delivery knowing their reward is not at all what they have been dreaming about. The swollen breasts that follow do not know that there is no baby there to suckle. Nature can be so unkind.

I was wishing I were somewhere else, but I sensed the woman needed a calming, caring heart. Mine is caring to a fault. This happened 20 years ago, but it seems like yesterday. I held her hand as her cervix began to dilate past six centimeters and she felt like pushing. There was no cheerleading. No "come on, you can do it, your baby is almost here!" No, just a quiet voice, my voice, telling her to push, that it was almost over. I sensed in her denial, that until she'd seen her still baby's body she wouldn't be convinced. I understood and felt the same way myself. As the head crowned, the doctor came in to attend the delivery. The dread was palpable. We all felt it. Had she had this baby four days earlier, we would be shouting, but this time luck was not on her side. It was two days ago when she felt the last kick. We put her legs in stirrups, did the proper prep, and had all the instruments in order. There was little talking, only a quiet concentration to get this over with. As the doctor maneuvered the baby's head to release the anterior shoulder, I was suddenly frightened that he was inadvertently pulling the head too hard. It looked as though the two or three days of floating in fluid might cause this poor baby's head to come off. Yes, it happens sometimes. Thank God not this time. "One more push!" I said. The baby slid out lifeless. I realized I was actually holding my breath. I saw my patient look down ever so briefly. "Would you like to hold your baby?" I asked. She hesitated. I told her I would clean her beautiful little daughter up and swaddle her in blankets. She relented and said under her breath, "Okay."

As I was carrying the baby and weighing her delicate, perfect body, she was a sturdy six pounds, eight ounces. A full-size, fully formed baby.

Too heavy in my mind to not be crying, to not protest as I poked and prodded at her. I had to be extra careful while wrapping her. Her skin was starting to peel away as the soft baby blanket rubbed against her.

I brought my dear patient her beautiful term infant, swaddled in a blanket, and carefully lay the baby in her arms. I cried as I looked at them. She finally cried, too. In just my ordinary eight-hour shift, I had become a different person. I was profoundly and forever changed. I will never forget my experience, or that patient. I know we connected on a deep level.

My shift came to an end. I clocked out and drove home faster than usual. I wanted to see my own six-month-old daughter asleep in her crib.

Several weeks later I received a gift at work. It was a pink jacket for me. How odd! I thought. Then I read the card and the tears started flowing once again. The patient was thanking me for taking such good care of her. I could hardly believe it. This young woman would thank *me*? Nurses, I believe, do more than tasks—we touch people and they touch our hearts. Forever.

Memoirs from an "Angel of Mercy"

~

Heather Tempest, RN, PNC(c)

ONE OF THE greatest miracles is that of bringing life into the world. As a seasoned labor and delivery nurse, I have seen many miracles and shared in many smiles, and many tears of joy, over the years. I have also shared in those experiences that evoke tears of sorrow, when for unknown reasons, the expected arrival is not meant to be or comes to an abrupt end.

I had the experience of being the nurse for a special woman who was expecting twins. I had known this woman indirectly prior to her pregnancy and knew the trials and heartaches she had endured over the years as she and her husband attempted to start a family. She had struggled through many attempts to maintain a pregnancy. As this pregnancy progressed and through stringent monitoring of her babies, it became apparent early in her final trimester that one of the twins would be stillborn. This wonderful couple had struggled through the very sensitive decision, after successful in-vitro treatments, to "reduce" a quadruplet pregnancy to that of twins, in hopes of protecting the two remaining babies. Now there was renewed fear that the remaining baby might be compromised as well. We started on what would prove an emotional roller coaster. There was a special bond that developed between this family and myself from this point and through delivery of the babies. This special bond would stay strong for many years thereafter. This was a woman in need of much emotional support, as she dealt with many conflicting emotions—emotions of sadness and joy.

As the day for her scheduled cesarean section approached, I rallied much support for her and her husband. We had spoken at length ahead of time about what to expect, how they would be able to hold both their children (two little girls) and spend time with them both together and separately, as they wished. There are no rules when offering the tender loving care needed for these couples. I also had arranged for support both from the hospital's chaplain and their own minister to be available as the family desired. I encouraged them to deal with each event in turn, and assured them that the nurses would be there to support whatever decisions they made along their journey.

I took a very nervous couple to the operating room that day and never left their side. We shared tears both before and during the surgery, as the woman clung to me throughout. Her husband, while trying to be stoic and supportive for his wife's sake, was quiet and subdued while the surgery was in progress. Being of European descent, he felt he needed to keep his emotions in check. As the little girls were delivered, I tenderly wrapped each wee bundle in a colorful blanket, placing a pink hat on one and a green hat on the other. One of the most poignant moments of the whole day was that first cry from Stephanie and then the stark silence in the room as the doctor handed me little Emily. The tears were flowing freely as I handed very relieved parents their beautiful daughter to cradle and held the beautiful stillborn myself.

During her recovery period, secluded in a sun-filled birthing suite away from the hustle of the busy unit, I took photographs, placed footprints of both girls, and snipped a lock of hair for the parents to treasure. We took pictures of the babies together and alone, as well as with their parents. I had encouraged the mom and dad to bring in their own camera as well that day. I allowed them to dictate what photographs they wished to have as meaningful mementos. A memory package in a beautiful white eyelet envelope was assembled, so that one day they might share this special day with the "living sister." There was so much emotion in the room that day that I left many hours later with a true sense of pride, accomplishment, and satisfaction. As a nurse, I had offered this family something special. The impact of this experience has benefited me in dealing with the many bereaved families I have cared for in my numerous years as an obstetrical nurse. Experiences such as this add true meaning to the words tender loving care—the special care that nurses are so known to give.

This very special patient went on to have a successful pregnancy and birth a few years following the birth of her twins. I felt honored to have developed such a special bond with this family. It allowed me to offer my support and understanding through yet another very emotionally charged and rocky pregnancy. I followed her through her trials, tears, and fears, from the very early stage of the pregnancy up to being her nurse the day of the birth. I experienced a rare relationship and felt proud to have been given the opportunity to offer my clinical wisdom, along with the element of human touch that nurses are known to provide with such expertise.

I again was present to see her and her husband through the day of her repeat cesarean section. On this important day, I wore an "angel" in honor of the twin that we all knew was dear to her parents' hearts. I also pinned an angel to her gown, to give her strength in the remembrance of those miracles that we never ever forget. On this day, we had returned to share in happy memories together.

After a successful surgery, little Natalie came into the world with a gusty howl, along with locks of red hair! On this occasion we shared many a happy tear, as well as a special remembrance for the darling little angel who shone down on her family that day. Angels live forever and will always be in the hearts of those who love them.

PART THREE

Supporting Parents

When a Baby's Short Life Is at Home

~

Cara Bicking, *RN, BSN*

For the first couple of years I worked in the neonatal intensive care unit, I was afraid to take care of babies who were going to die. I knew how to take care of the babies, but the families seemed to need so much more than I thought I could give them. As I grow as a nurse, however, I find that this reluctance is changing.

One particular morning I discovered that a four-day-old infant I had taken care of over the weekend would be sent home that day with comfort care, as his parents had chosen not to continue curative medicine. Although I saw some nurses cringe at the decision, I jumped at the opportunity to support this family's choice and requested the assignment for my 12-hour shift.

The infant, a full-term cutie named Joshua, had been transferred to our hospital for evaluation. He was presumed to have a rare syndrome that affects bone growth and is associated with cardiac defects. Prognosis depends on associated defects and Joshua suffered from a hole in his heart and lungs that had not developed at all, making his prognosis very poor. He was given a lot of extra oxygen through prongs in his nose but still did not always do very well. The infant was the fourth child born to Mennonite parents who had known before he was born of his diagnosis. The mother described her surprise when he had "come out screaming," as they had expected him to die soon after birth.

On the day of Joshua's discharge, I received report from the night-shift nurse, who told me that Joshua would go home with his parents using tube feedings and far more oxygen than was generally given to NICU babies. She also said that the IV catheter going into Joshua's umbilical vein was to be removed in the morning, and that she had strict orders not to give him any intravenous medication because he wouldn't have an IV at home. The nurse did report that she had to give the infant one dose of IV Versed during the night for agitation. I knew from my previous time with Joshua that he occasionally became very agitated, presumably because it was very hard for him to breathe. He had often been inconsolable and normal things like holding, rocking, and swaddling did not help to calm him.

After report was over, Joshua again became extremely irritable, and he turned blue because his sick heart and lungs couldn't keep up with the demands that crying put on his little body. I immediately approached the attending physician, knowing that the resident physicians would have no ability to overturn his decisions, and inquired about giving medication to help relieve Joshua's discomfort. Although the attending was at first reluctant to offer any solution, I pointed out that the infant could not go home to be with his family on the basis of providing comfort if he was constantly miserable. I felt very strongly about advocating for the comfort of this baby, who in all likelihood felt that he was suffocating to death. The attending said, "I don't know what we can give him." I politely told him that not knowing just wasn't an option. As a nurse, it's our job to stand up to physicians and press on for the welfare of the patient. Eventually we were able to collaborate with the pediatric pharmacist and discovered that Versed can also be given under the baby's tongue. The order was written to trial this method with the infant.

In continuing discharge planning for the newborn, I had the parents give him a bath and dress him. I taught them how to insert the feeding tube and the father performed this task beautifully. Joshua's mother then held him while his father prepared and administered the feeding. Joshua was calmed by the administration of Versed, and I spoke extensively with the family about their view of their baby's need for medication. I thought they might prefer comfort measures over medication because of their Mennonite culture, but they felt Joshua was very uncomfortable and that they could not help him without the medication. I told them when he would need the Versed and how often they could give it to him, recognizing and communicating that his comfort was more important than strictly adhering to the rules of giving his medication only every two hours. In the hospital, so much depends on strictly following the rules and orders in order to make a baby healthy. In preparing a baby to go home to be with his family at the end of life, a big lesson I learned as a nurse is that the rules can be bent to serve the needs of the baby and the family.

While the infant's father stepped out of the NICU to visit the pharmacy, I sat in a rocking chair next to the baby and his mother and had a long, quiet conversation with her. I wanted to create an environment where she would be comfortable confiding in me and discussing her fears so that some of her anxiety could be reduced. We discussed her feelings about Joshua's care, his comfort, her family's reaction to his birth and homecoming, and her fears about him being at home. She was focused on allowing her baby to be at home with his family, even if it lasted only a short while. I also spoke to her extensively about the signs Joshua might show when his heart stopped working as effectively or when his lungs could no longer compensate as well as they did at the time and explained the physiologic reason for each symptom. I felt it was important for her to be aware of the signs and symptoms of heart failure so that she would know that the progression she observed was expected and would not need to be anxious or think that something drastic might happen at any moment. Joshua's mother thanked me for this information, saying that she might have been very frightened to see these changes in her baby, but now that she understood, she "wouldn't be so freaked out." I also debated whether to tell her how I felt about their decision for their baby's care, but finally told her that I felt that they had made the right choice for Joshua and their family by taking him home to be cared for. She actually breathed an audible sigh of relief. I think that although she believed their decision was right, any parents would question themselves, and she needed to hear that a caring medical professional also thought they were doing the right thing.

As our conversation came to an end, I employed a technique I learned in one of my master's-level classes in order to be sure that the parents' questions had been answered and that they would be comfortable with their child's care. I asked the baby's mother to tell me what she thought the first day at home would be like for Joshua and her family, and to take me step-by-step through the process of the day. Her description uncovered questions about cleaning Joshua's feeding supplies and when to call the physician. This technique is wonderful for identifying issues of practicality that otherwise wouldn't be thought about until the baby is already home.

When Joshua's parents had been taught all aspects of his care and had run out of questions, we prepared to discharge him. Joshua, his parents, the attending physician, and I left the unit with three bags of supplies and two enormous oxygen tanks. As I waited with Joshua's mother inside the hospital entrance with the baby for the men to load the transport van, she turned and thanked me for all I had done to help her family. She was very emotional and said, "You're the best nurse we've had here; thank you so much for everything." I was touched deeply by her sincerity. Before departure Joshua's father also thanked me just as sincerely, and I knew by the looks on their faces that the help I had provided them had enabled their son to die at home with his family. I knew this meant everything to this family and that by advocating for their baby's comfort, teaching them his care, and providing emotional support, I had been able to have a positive impact on a family in crisis.

I later found out that Joshua had died at home the very next morning. The parents had told me earlier in their hospital stay that the thing they were most afraid of was having their baby die in the hospital. There was nothing more rewarding than knowing that a family dealing with the tragedy of the loss of their newborn son could be comforted by the work of their nurse and the other health-care professionals who had all worked together to make their wishes for his life come true.

Circle of Life

~

Kelly Maidment, RN

THE TEAM IS at the ready—nurses, respiratory therapists, and a neonatology resident. The doorway to Room A is open, giving way to the adjacent labor and delivery suites. The night outside is dark and quiet. Inside, the fluorescent lights hum and there is a flurry of activity in preparation for the arrival of our new guest. Equipment is prepared—intubations tray is on standby, as well as a ventilator. The element of the over-bed warmer glows orange and hot. Intravenous solutions are warming and hearing the swoosh of a green hospital gown, we know that our guest is now traversing the halls in the arms of one of the NICU nurses and about to arrive in our unit.

I can't remember what time or date it was. All the nights blur together with a certain sameness, and yet there are some that lodge themselves in our mind, that become embedded whether we want them to or not. Despite the fact that names and faces and often specific details may seem blurred or faded like a memory from an old photograph, we will experience events and emotions here that will stay with us for a lifetime. A tattoo on our memory, our very psyche. We all experience things that affect us in ways that run deeply. What begins as just another mundane work night can end up being something that echoes in the reaches of your heart and mind, changing you for the better, or perhaps for the worse.

The newest guest to our 28-bed Level III neonatal intensive care unit is placed under the bright lights of the warmer bed, dried, and placed in a sterile bag to prevent heat loss. Cardiac monitors are applied, oxygen sensor is on, the baby is suctioned, weighed, and intubated, surfactant is given, central lines are inserted. Fluids are started, X-rays performed. Blood work is drawn and sent, antibiotics are started. Happy birthday, baby. What a party you have had! Welcome to the world as you know it.

All has gone well in this baby's resuscitation and in two hours, give or take, the newest guest in our unit is ready to meet his parents for the first time after his arrival this night. The doctor had already been in to update the parents on their baby's condition. They are aware that their son is a micro-perm. His gestation is about 26 weeks. His prognosis: long road ahead, with the potential for many pitfalls and no guarantees. He could have cerebral palsy, blindness, deafness, or learning delays—if, that is, he doesn't succumb to infection, necrotizing entercolitis, intraventricular hemorrhage, or any of the other problems this fragile person may have to overcome. With all our technology and our medical advances we still can't offer guarantees, but at least he has a chance and there is hope. However, the harsh reality is that this baby and ones like him have a long, hard fight ahead of them.

Before he is settled in his humidified incubator, his parents come to meet their new son. Their firstborn child. A son they never planned to meet so soon and under such circumstances. A child that must look alien to them with his gelatinous-looking skin and large head, and with the number of wires and tubes running to and from his small frame. His grief-stricken mother cannot control her pain and she is overwrought with a torrent of emotions at the sight of her helpless baby. Her body shudders when she sees the child who only hours ago lived protected within her womb. She blames herself, as so many do, for his untimely arrival. Dad tries to remain calm and stoic, but it is evident that he is blinking back tears that are stinging his weary, bloodshot eyes. After a brief visit and orientation to the unit and the equipment that is helping to support their son (most of which they are too stressed and tired to retain at this point), they take their leave so that an exhausted postpartum mother can be settled in her room and she, too, can receive the care that she needs. As she is settled in, her son is settled in his incubator. Thus far, this is quite a typical shift in our unit. Nothing remarkable. This is what we do. It's the first shift during which I cared for this baby. What makes me remember my first shift with this baby is the second shift that I took care of him.

I walked in to get my assignment, and the nurse in charge looked up with a grimace and said, "Sorry." No "Hi, how are you?"; just "sorry." That is never a good way to start off a shift and is usually a strong indicator of one thing. After approximately one month of severe pulmonary issues and feeding intolerances and a tiny body ravaged by infection, it was clear that the baby could no longer take any more, and the excruciating decision was made by his parents to withdraw the support of the machines that were artificially prolonging the life of their little boy. I had cared for this baby on the night of his birth and so now, on the night of his death. This is the part of my job that people don't often ask about. Perhaps because they feel it is a taboo subject or perhaps because it does not occur to them, but it happens. This is a harsh reality of being a nurse in the neonatal intensive care unit. Babies sometimes die. It is something you never get use to. I'm guessing that if you do, it is time to find a new profession because you have officially reached burnout capacity. Certainly, we as nurses must learn to maintain a certain degree of professional composure and ability to compartmentalize. This is self-preservation, but the moment the wails of a mother cradling her newly deceased baby stop affecting you, it's time to move on. I have yet to burn out. Every time a baby dies, I still get a sick and sinking feeling in my stomach and I hurt for these families.

This night the decision has been made. The papers have been signed and the parents are already cuddling their little one in a private family room. His breathing tube has been removed and his life hangs precariously in the balance. With each passing minute, his young life draws closer to its end. It is now a waiting game as to how long he can hold on without the assistance of our machines, of how much strength his young, frail body has left. I check in with the family periodically to offer them support and what little comfort I can, and to check his heart rate. I explain to the parents that their son's breathing may change, becoming irregular and eventually slowing to a halt. They understand, and I try to prepare them for what is fast approaching. They understand. They understand that his tiny heart will slow and eventually stop, and in this quiet, softly lift room, their little boy will leave them. Peacefully, quietly, and without suffering. They know that they as parents have done everything they could for their son and that their decision was the right one. They have begun to show acceptance in this process, and the sobs have subsided into quiet tears and contemplation.

I once again take my leave so that they might be a family again for a few minutes without the intrusion of what equates to a near stranger. I sit outside the door of the family room and wait for when I am needed.

Twenty minutes later the father emerges. "Can you check?" he says, pale and gaunt. He knows. I bring my stethoscope in and listen to a tiny silent chest. I get the neonatalgist to confirm what we all already know. Their tiny son has tired. His reserve is depleted and he has let go. Their son is gone. There is much sadness, but I think there is also relief, as they know their child no longer suffers. Over the next hour, they cuddle and kiss and say their final good-byes. I can only imagine what this is like for these parents. Trying to burn every tiny detail into their mind's eyes lest they ever forget a feel, a smell, a trait that their baby has. Trying to hold onto the feeling of a baby that will never know the touch of their hands again. The pain must be insurmountable. It is truly heartbreaking.

When the parents finally feel ready to go, they emerge, mother swaddling her precious bundle in her arms, father supporting her in his. He gives me a weak smile, as does his wife. She stares lovingly down at her baby and squeezes him tightly to her engorged bosom, which is now full and heavy with milk she no longer needs. This is their final good-bye. The father gently and softly tells her, "It's okay, let Suzanna take care of him now," and with that she hands me her son, already cold and dark. They turn and walk away together. They are spent and weak and full of a pain only someone who has experienced this loss can imagine. And I am left standing there, holding what was once the most precious thing in the world to these people. They have entrusted me this night with his care as they had a month or so ago, which to all of us seems like a lifetime ago. In fact it was a lifetime ago—this baby's. The night on which his circle of life had begun, so, too, had it ended.

As nurses we have a unique and profound ability to have an impact on the people around us, and inversely, we feel their impact. We gain insight into the tremendous ability that the human animal has for strength and resilience, to be compassionate, and to love and be loved. And as drops of water have the strength to forge a valley through a mountain, these tiny babies, the smallest population in our health care system, can leave the most profound and lasting impact on the lives of those they touch, even if their circle is small.

Better Late Than Never

~

Dawn M. Kersula, MA, RN, FACCE, IBCLC

SHE BROUGHT THE sunshine into the room when she walked into class. I'm an experienced Lamaze teacher, so I breathed a sigh of relief as she asked all the questions I hoped she'd ask: What is labor really like? Can women's bodies really give birth to a baby without drugs? Will my husband be tough enough to stay with me?

He was a hockey player. Everybody knew them—they'd been high school sweethearts, and the other students in Lamaze class seemed to think some of the sunshine and the glory would rub off, just being able to hobnob with them in class. I just thanked my lucky stars that they were eager, intelligent, totally in love with each other and this new adventure in their life together, and willing to learn.

Each week in class, I would weave a vision of the future that included breastfeeding their babies. After all, our hospital breastfeeding initiation rate was over 90 percent, and in the community "everybody" breastfeeds. Because I felt so strongly about breastfeeding, and struggled with my own feelings about women who chose to formula-feed their babies, I never asked who was planning to do what. It worked well to imagine each one of "my moms" breastfeeding happily—and to tell the truth, I was seldom disappointed.

The class "graduated," with promises of support and happy reunions. Birthing days quickly came for each couple. And the golden couple became a mom and dad—a happy birth, straightforward and drug-free, produced a beautiful and healthy baby boy.

When I came in to work the next day, I was dismayed. My golden girl and her darling baby—not breastfeeding? Well, people make their own best choices. I could still congratulate her and support her.

I walked into the room, and there he was, the next little hockey-playing generation. He and his mom were so in love, locked in that wondrous gaze, eye to eye, soul to soul. A sigh, a shrug, and he was off to sleep.

Want to try some skin-to-skin? She was an early child development major—you bet she'd like to try it! We turned the lights down low, took off her shirt, unwrapped her sleep-drunk son, and placed him between her breasts. The look on her face was one of naked, unmasked love.

The baby snuggled in. She began to cry. "Oh, this is so wonderful! I love him so much!"

Suddenly his little body churned into action. As we watched, he hurtled down to her right breast—and began to suckle!

The world seemed to stand still.

After what seemed like a lifetime, she looked up at me, her eyes glistening and sparkling. "I guess he knew what he wanted. He already knows how to breastfeed."

As I left the room, I must admit to a moment of self-satisfaction, but I was also floored by the competence and determination of this great little guy.

Pulled that one right out of the bag! I thought to myself.

I looked forward to seeing them the next day. I was devastated to hear that she had decided not to continue breastfeeding. My Lamaze classes always love to have new parents come and talk to them, and the golden couple and their lovely less-than-optimally fed baby came and clearly showed the joys of attachment parenting—holding your baby as much as possible, keeping close even at night, attending to the baby's needs. They grew and prospered.

Fast-forward three years, and the couple came back, pregnant with their second son. An older couple in the community had given them a great deal on a house, First Son was a delightful preschooler, and Golden Girl was working in Early Head Start. It was great to see that their life continued to be blessed, but I still felt sad that she was a formula feeder.

"Hey Dawn . . . I've been learning for the past three years about all the good things about breastfeeding. Will you help me breastfeed this baby?"

You bet I would—and her attachment parenting skills made it very easy for her new little son to breastfeed. She knew her babies, she knew herself, and Hockey Dad glowed with pride because he now enjoyed a skating three-year-old and a new boy to teach.

Three years later, Golden Girl was directing the Home Visitors Program at Early Education Services. She teaches other teachers how to help with breastfeeding—because she has become a certified lactation counselor herself! And some of the teaching came from her *third* baby, born with health challenges but wonderfully loved and breastfed.

You'll still see her today—she's the perky gal with caramel hair, with all the moms and kids around her at the Pee Wee hockey games. She glows with vitality and love—and her daughter is learning hockey, too.

How many women will decide to try breastfeeding because of their love and willingness to try something new? I can't tell. But I know that when I asked her after Baby Three, "Why did you come late to breastfeeding?" her reply was, "I never knew anyone who breastfed. I needed to learn how wonderful it was."

These days I still see every mom as a potential nursing mother, strong and wonderful, and I am seldom disappointed.

Ayub: A Parent's Story of Fear, Love, and Determination

~

Suzanna M. Feliciano,
BSN, RN, CCRN

Ayub was born the summer of 2008 at 37 5/7 weeks' gestation with a rare birth defect: septo-optic dysplasia (de Morsier syndrome). Such a beautiful baby boy, but so many broken dreams for this young couple. This was their first child. Every parent wants to hear the words "what a beautiful baby." But when mom and the maternal grandmother were given the devastating news, their only response was, "It can't be!"

Seeing this mother cry with such emotion left a great impression on my heart that morning. Further testing was scheduled to confirm these findings. This beautiful baby boy appears normal on the outside. He has all his fingers and toes, his head is nice and round, he has a beautiful smooth skin color and moves all his extremities, but he is quiet and does not feed well. His rare disorder is a condition involving the triad of optic nerve hypoplasia (ONH), midline brain abnormality, and pituitary hypoplasia with subsequent endocrine dysfunction.

This is a story about the fear, hope, and determination of a young couple. Their new baby boy has multiple problems: galactosemia, optic nerve dysplasia, diabetes insipidus (DI), pituitary deficiency, and absence of septum pellucidum.

Baby Ayub was delivered by spontaneous vaginal delivery after artificial rupture of membranes without complications and transitioned to Nursery Level I. On his first day of life he fed poorly, with a very weak suck reflex, and developed hyperbilirubinemia.

He was transferred to our Level II care (the neonatal intensive care unit) so that the medical staff could begin intravenous fluids, draw further lab values, evaluate for sepsis, and begin phototherapy. Repeat bilirubin continued to show elevation. By his third day of life, signs of improvement were slow and he was still feeding poorly. His first neonatal screen had detected probable galactosemia. His formula was changed to soy base. There were no signs of cardiac or respiratory compromise. Our faculty neonatologist ordered a head ultrasound to be performed at the bedside. More bad news: There is no septum pellucidum! More laboratory tests were sent: levels for ADH, cortical, testosterone, thyroid stimulating hormone (TSH), growth hormone, and chromosome studies.

An MRI was performed and confirmed the diagnoses. Ophthalmology had examined and also confirmed optic nerve hypoplasia. After all the information was collected, our faculty physician and neonatal nurse practitioner reported this information to the mom and maternal grandmother. As would be expected, both were devastated by the final conclusions. Realizing that the baby would have pituitary gland dysfunction, we upgraded baby Ayub to Level III care.

I was privileged to begin discharge teaching and educate the family on the clinical manifestations associated will the diagnoses. Realizing that this child would be going home on multiple medications, my first goal was to educate the parents about each associated problem. Our hospital system allows employees access to a database for research on medical and nursing issues. This allowed me to share articles and information with the parents. Ayub is unique, because there were not any reported cases identical to his. Most similar cases have one or two of the clinical problems, but Ayub's case involves neurological, endocrine, and physical symptoms.

I began by educating the parents on the associated endocrine problems: delayed growth, developmental delay, hypothyroidism, hypoglycemia, lethargy, pituitary hormone deficiency, and ocular dysfunction with unknown visual impairment. The dad was fluent in English, but the mom preferred instruction in Spanish. This would be a challenge for the entire medical and nursing team. Initially, the mom would come in, hold her baby, and ask questions like, "Is he stable?" or "What is his weight today?" She was hearing some things, but not everything. Although I am bilingual, there are many medical terms that I don't use day after day, so frequently I access a translator site from the web to facilitate my teaching to parents.

At this phase, the parents and extended family were still experiencing shock and disbelief at all the information they had been given by our medical team. It is a blessing for these young parents to have such a great family support system. Both maternal and paternal grandmothers were present throughout the hospital period and were available to help their children through this difficult time and until they were discharged to their home. I was able to communicate with this family very well. I understood their cultural concerns, and I was able to speak frankly with both parents about the importance of their role in understanding and learning about their baby's problems so they could help him maximize all his potentials as he grew. I reminded them that they needed to be very attentive to his behaviors, his overall hydration, and his developmental milestones. They would be the first to detect deficits, and they needed to seek assistance immediately before there was any progression of problems. I also remember telling the mom in front of her mother-in-law that she needed to keep an open heart and mind if her family recognized something in her baby as he grew that might not seem "normal." I reminded her about a Spanish phrase that translates to "don't shut yourself from the world around you." Her mother-in-law replied, "You see, that's what we told you."

Oftentimes as professionals we need to be more direct, and this can be a very effective method to teach when stress is high and the attention span is short. Repetition and continuity of care were important to teach these parents; it helped them feel empowered, and we gained their trust. The endocrine service was consulted to join the neonatal team. Together they reviewed all the data, examined the baby, and met the mom.

My second discharge goal was focused on teaching the parents how to administer injections to their baby. We had just begun subcutaneous injection of DDAVP (Desmopressin acetate), 0.04 micrograms SQ every 12 hours. The medical team recommended a class for the parents at our Diabetic Teaching Clinic. The parents received instructions on dosage calculation and intramuscular injection of cortisone, should their baby experience a stressful situation or become acutely ill. They attended this class and obtained instructional material in Spanish. When they completed this session, they could acknowledge the difference between IM and SQ. They expressed how grateful they were for all the attention we were giving them. It was a joy working with this young couple during this first intense week. I continued to provide them information about their child's disease and a list of resources and web links for future reading. I also created a personalized daily schedule that included oral medications and the injections.

By the second week, their confidence had increased. They were asking more questions and had forgotten some of their fears. I scheduled the injections of DDAVP so they could share the responsibility according to their schedule. The mother came in by 9 A.M. and dad came in at 9 P.M. I would have them check each other as they drew up the medication and then verify it with me or the night nurse. It was such a tiny dose to measure and when I first showed them that it was just two drops, they realized how potent it must be.

Another portion of our teaching process involved measuring urine output. Early on, baby Ayub developed signs of diabetes insipidus and was placed on a vasopressin infusion and later converted to DDAVP injections every 12 hours. Our discharge nurse obtained a diaper scale. I taught the parents how to weigh diapers and start learning how to evaluate the effectiveness of DDAVP on urine output. We reviewed the signs and symptoms of dehydration. I purchased a small binder and instructed the parents to keep a record of urine output and formula intake so they could see the response of DDAVP. I reminded them this would be a good method to learn how to dose this medication as their child grew and to help their doctor adjust the medication.

What a great experience this was for me! This young couple accepted the responsibility that their son would be on hormone replacement therapy for the rest of his life. He would require comprehensive eye exams, genetic counseling, long-term follow-up with a neurologist and endocrinologist, and physical therapy. I am still impressed with this young couple. In spite of all the problems they faced, they took charge and learned how to care for their baby.

The first few days after discharge, the parents called several times for reassurance. We encourage all our parents to call our unit and our medical team for any questions or concerns, especially if they have not had their pediatrician appointment. The first week home was the most difficult for them. They had two emergency room visits when they feared dehydration or increased urination. Today, one month later, they are doing great and are very confident.

PART FOUR

When Nurses Bond

Baby Jamie, Who I Promise Not to Forget…

~

Carol Blair-Murdoch, RN, BSCN

SITTING ON MY windowsill along with many family photos is a small Winnie-the-Pooh frame with a smiling baby boy and a quote on the back reading "Promise you won't forget me, ever. Not even when I'm a hundred." I have not forgotten him and will share our story.

I am astonished at how quickly time has passed since my early days of nursing, the travels and the special people I have been blessed to meet and the impact they have had on my life. It was 19 years ago that I returned to my position at the Hospital for Sick Children's Cardiology unit from an exciting leave of absence, which included a three-month nursing locum in a neonatal intensive care unit in Saudi Arabia followed by six months of backpacking through Asia. Within a few weeks, I resettled into the routine and hectic pace of the cardiology unit and was assigned to a very special baby boy that to this day I remember with love.

He was the first baby that I cared for who was the happy result of in vitro fertilization, which at the time—in 1989—was rather special. He proved to be "special" in more ways than one as our relationship developed. Despite being a newborn, he had undergone his first heart surgery to begin to address a complex congenital heart lesion. For being so young he had already been through a great deal. He had an incision that was not healing well and required deep moist packing and dressing changes. It was the one part of him that healed slowly despite meticulous nursing care.

In pediatric nursing, a bond is established with both the child and the parent. In Jamie's case, I really clicked with the whole family. Jamie's mother was an intensive care nurse from England who worked and lived with her Canadian husband in Bermuda. We all loved to travel and talked at length about our adventures, in addition to caring for our lovely boy, who was airlifted from their tiny island to Toronto for heart surgery shortly after birth. When his dad returned to work, I developed a very close friendship with his mother and his grandmother, who flew over for support. I remember convincing Jamie's mom to leave the hospital for one evening to join my family at Thanksgiving dinner. We had a lovely evening talking with my parents and grandparents about England, Bermuda, and of course

Jamie. She enjoyed the break from the hospital and joined us again for another family dinner.

As Jamie's core nurse, I rode the emotional roller coaster with his parents as his condition worsened, improved, and then finally worsened again as the fall season progressed. I took care of Jamie every shift I worked. I knew how to comfort him and make him smile, when he was well enough. His mother laughingly suggested his first word might in fact be "Carol," which of course is my name.

I admired his mother tremendously. She did everything she could with love to encourage and facilitate Jamie's healing. She went to great lengths, providing him with increased-calorie breast milk using a small tube attached to her breast as he breastfed. We then would supplement the rest through his nasogastric tube. She continued breastfeeding throughout Jamie's ups and downs, with the help of a lactation consultant and supportive nurses, until he was no longer able to take his feedings by mouth.

His cardiac condition was unfortunately worsening, and he required a second, more complex, surgery. By late November, Jamie was back in the intensive care unit in an incredibly unstable postoperative state. His nursing care was now out of my hands. Like his mother, I too was overwhelmed with his status, the supports he required, and my lack of control. He began to change in appearance due to the swelling that occurs from numerous fluid boluses to maintain blood pressure in a body where the heart and kidneys begin to fail. He was pharmaceutically muscle relaxed with a sternum left open due to swelling, and had numerous drains and intravenous lines carrying a great deal of cardiovascular support medications. Images of him smiling at us seemed so long ago.

Fortunately, he had core nurses in the intensive care unit as well. One in particular cared for him very regularly, as I did on the ward. She even worked overtime shifts near the end of his life to continue to care for him at his most critical time. It was different back then with respect to "circle of care," and she shared information with me freely as a colleague and family support. I was part of his Canadian family. Many of us were.

Earlier on in the year, I had booked a trip to New Zealand to visit friends I had met while backpacking in Asia. I was scheduled to fly on December 29. It was getting close to Christmastime, and Jamie was in a very critical state. He passed away in the presence of his mom, dad, and various core nurses shortly before my trip. I will never forget getting that call from the hospital. There was a horrible snowstorm and I was unable to get there. I was devastated and was unable to contemplate my travel plans. Unfortunately, however, there was no renegotiating the ticket with the airline. Jamie's mom and my family encouraged me to stick with my original plans and I left the next day.

As I was flying to New Zealand, Jamie and his family flew to England, where he was buried near his grandfather. There was a service held at the Hospital for Sick Children for the staff who loved and cared for him, as attending the funeral in England was not an option. I appreciated the fact that the nursing management acknowledged what a loss this was for many of us.

To this day, I cherish my memories of him and keep his small photo with my special family photos on the windowsill. He has a special place in my heart. Despite living in different countries, I have kept in touch with his family over the years. Today they are proud and loving parents of teenage triplets! I had the pleasure of meeting them when they were toddlers in Bermuda and again as preteens in England. They visited Canada four years ago when my son was born. His mom shared privately with me that she appreciated the love I shared with her first son and was pleased that I now had a boy of my own to love.

David's Miracle

∾

Lanette L. Anderson, MSN, JD, RN

Oₙₑ ᴏꜰ ᴛʜᴇ most wonderful things about the nursing profession is the wide variety of options that are available in terms of careers. We can provide care to patients and families in many types of settings. We can also research, teach, publish, and work as legal nurse consultants. The opportunities seem almost endless.

I have not been involved in clinical practice for several years, as my career has gravitated toward an emphasis on nursing regulation, administrative law, and the education of bachelor and master of science in nursing students. I often miss the clinical setting, and wonder what it would be like to return to the bedside. My specialty area is neonatal intensive care nursing, which is a world unlike any other. I have so many memories of my years in NICU. I cherish the happy memories and learned much from the heartbreaking experiences that unfortunately come with the territory.

I'll never forget David. It was a 12-hour night shift (my third in a row), and I had been assigned to get any new admissions for that shift. The assignment of new admissions itself was stressful; you hoped that you received no new babies but prepared for the worst-case scenario. Preparation was both mental and physical. I had to pay attention to what was going on in Labor and Delivery, and also make sure that if a new arrival came to the NICU, I had a fully stocked bed ready.

At around 11:30 PM, an orderly from the emergency room walked casually into the NICU carrying blankets and what I initially presumed was a stillbirth for us to weigh and measure. As I approached him to see what he needed, I saw a tiny hand waving amidst the blankets. Prior to his arrival, I was beginning to get sleepy; I quickly became alert. I immediately turned on a warming bed and monitors. I took the blankets and gently unwrapped them. Inside was a baby boy with bright red hair sticking up all over his head. I began assessing him with the help of my co-workers. His temperature was dangerously low. He was small, approximately four pounds, but appeared to be full term. He cried weakly, but did not appear to be in any respiratory distress. His oxygen saturation was adequate; however, his glucose level was also very low. I turned on extra warming lights and started an IV to administer glucose, antibiotics, and whatever else he might need.

After the initial stabilization of the baby, we began to notice other things about him that were concerning. In addition to his being small for gestational age, his facial features were unusual. His face was somewhat flat, his lips were small, and his head was small. I realized that we had not received much history about this new baby, other than that he had been born at home. My next job was to attempt to learn as much as I could about his short life prior to his arrival in the NICU.

The next few hours were frustrating. The emergency room staff initially could not tell me much, as the baby's mother apparently was not cooperating with their questioning. The significant other who had accompanied her to the ER also wasn't talking. Even getting information about the age of the mother was difficult, as she gave several different ages ranging from mid-20s to early 50s. Her stories about how, when, and where the delivery occurred also changed. One constant about working NICU is that just when you think you have heard everything, something else comes in the door. After getting a report from the emergency medical technicians who had responded to the 911 call and brought her and the baby to the ER, we learned information that was difficult to hear and more difficult to cognitively process.

David had indeed been born at home, to a mother in her late 40s. She was intoxicated at the time of labor and delivery, as was the significant other. After the birth, he tied the cord with a shoelace and cut it with a razor blade. It was difficult to determine how much time passed before they decided to call 911, but the delay undoubtedly was the cause of David's hypothermia and hypoglycemia.

David was his mother's sixth child. All five others had been removed from her custody by Child Protective Services. The fifth child, a girl, had been found alone in a car outside the apartment where she lived while she was drunk inside. As I looked at this sweet child, I knew that we as nurses had a huge challenge on our hands.

I telephoned the neonatologist on call and let him know about the situation. He arrived in the NICU within just a few minutes. He looked at David without saying a word, then went out to the desk and returned with a perinatology book. He turned the pages to a group of photos, looked at David, and looked back at the photos. After hearing the maternal history, his diagnosis was confirmed: David had full-blown fetal alcohol syndrome. He was likely to have long-term neurological damage.

Over the course of the next few days, I faced significant challenges. I had bonded with this baby and became his primary nurse. He initially seemed irritable and hypersensitive to touch, sound, and other stimuli. Eventually he became less resistant to physical contact, but he had a poor sucking reflex and feeding him was time-consuming. I held him every time that I had a spare few precious minutes.

In addition to his physical nursing care, which was fairly routine after his medical issues stabilized, dealing with his mother's behavior was a challenge like none I had previously experienced. She came to visit him daily.

Typically, she smelled of alcohol and appeared intoxicated. She urinated on the floor of the NICU on one occasion. Though she usually didn't ask to hold or feed David, she always talked about how she could not wait to get him home. I was proud of how I was able to remain professional and say basically nothing in response, when I really wanted to tell her that she would have to pry him out of my cold, dead hands before that happened. We all know that our role is to be nonjudgmental and practice therapeutic communication with our patients and families; however, in reality we have occasional thoughts that if expressed out loud would probably cost us our job. I am no exception.

Our unit staff worked closely with Social Services and Child Protective Services, so I was aware before the mother was that she would not take David home with her. I was not the individual who gave her this news, so I'm not sure how she reacted. My guess is that since this was not a new experience for her, she did not put up much resistance.

David was ultimately adopted by a wonderful couple. His father is a social worker, and his mother is a teacher. When I last heard, David was thriving and was developmentally and physically doing as well as could be expected. Although he may have learning disabilities, developmental delays, hyperactivity, or other long-term effects of fetal alcohol syndrome, I know that he is loved and nurtured. He is one of the most wonderful "success stories" that I have ever known. I'll never forget that bright red hair, that sweet face, and the true miracle that he survived at all.

PART FIVE

Lessons Learned

Stolen Time

~

Margie Marier-Porchia, *RN, BS*

ANOTHER DAY OF doing the job I love so much, and today is even better than usual. Today I get to do a Neonatal Individualized Developmental Care and Assessment Program observation of a baby. Doing a NIDCAP allows me to forget the tedious tasks of being a bedside nurse and gives me the opportunity to watch the infant. I watch the infant very closely, looking for any twitch, movement, or change in breathing or skin color. I am trying to listen to his body movements and his behaviors to help figure out what he is trying to say so that we can make things easier for him.

So the NIDCAP begins, and today is a little more stressful for me than usual. I am also being watched by my NIDCAP trainer and mentor. I aspire to her level of vision and sensitivity. We are watching the baby together to make sure I am seeing all of the same things she sees. With our clipboards and pencils in hand, ready to record his every movement, we begin.

This baby came into the world at just over 25 weeks' gestation and is now less than a day old. His mother's water broke several weeks ago, and she went into premature labor that could not be stopped. Weighing only one and a half pounds, he had a rough start, needing to be intubated and put on a breathing machine right after his birth. He required several medications and blood through special umbilical lines. Now receiving top medical care, he rests in a warm bed with a mist tent surrounding his body to protect his fragile skin. The lights in his room are dim, and the room is quiet except for the vibrating sound of his ventilator and an occasional alarm from his monitor. The nurse and respiratory therapist stand inches from his bed, watching him closely. His parents stand a few feet from the bed, talking quietly.

As the large machine barreled through the door, we realized it was time for his head ultrasound check. This is a fairly routine test to check a baby's brain for any bleeding or problems. As the technicians prepared their equipment, the nurse turned off the bright phototherapy light and moved it away from his bed. She lifted the mist tent that surrounded him and removed the goggles that covered his eyes. His dad took a quick picture; then the family moved farther from the bed and looked on. They stood close to each other, worried but relieved that he had done so well since his birth last night.

As the technician began the head ultrasound, he put a clear gel on the end of the instrument and placed it on the top of the infant's head. The infant appeared to be startled, moving his arms and legs and making a fist with his left hand. His movements caused his arms and legs to twitch and appear jittery. His forehead seemed to be trying to pull his eyes open, though they were fused. The nurse used her hands to tuck his arms and legs close to him and to try to calm him. He reached out with his right hand and grasped her finger, his tiny grasp barely making it around. The ultrasound tech finished the test after a few minutes and wiped the gel from the infant's head. The nurse replaced his eye covers and turned the bright light back on as she moved it closer to his bed. She was careful to place the mist tent back over him just right so she would not disturb the lines and tubing that surrounded him. The technicians left the room with their machine.

As I focused on watching how the infant would settle in after the activity, my mentor approached the family to give them a brief idea of our purpose there. We would be looking out for his developmental care and progress during his stay in the NICU. She told them their baby seemed to be responding to noises and stimulation and that we would keep his room quiet to help him rest. The family seemed thankful to have us on his side. They sat at his bedside for a few minutes, then left the room.

We systematically continued to record his responses during our intense observation. Though he seemed drowsy, over the next 15 minutes he twitched, extended his arms and legs outward, and made swallowing motions intermittently. He seemed to hear both sounds at his bedside and voices or alarms from an adjacent room. What was he trying to say? Was he simply responding to the noise and stimulation around him? Was he stressed?

The news came quickly. The head ultrasound showed a large area of bleeding in the left side of his brain. His outcome was very poor. The doctor shared the news with the parents, who agreed that keeping their baby alive was futile.

Immediately I knew that I had failed this little one. How could I be his voice if I did not listen to what he was saying? I had failed to realize what his true needs were. His needs were to feel his mother's touch and to hear his father's strong voice. While we were gathering data and making great plans for his care, we had denied his parents special moments. I had stolen precious time from this family. Instead of reporting on how he twitched and shook and struggled, I would have gladly set my clipboard and pencil down and watched him respond to his parents by grasping his mother's finger or turning his head toward his father's voice. Maybe if he'd had the chance to sense their presence more closely, he wouldn't have kicked his legs and struggled to open his eyes. His final outcome might have been the same, but during his short life he could have been comforted knowing that the bond he had with his parents was still ever present.

We can do a lot for infants, but promoting bonding and capturing special moments for families should be paramount in our priorities. We should take time when we have it, never missing the opportunity to help parents accept, love, and touch their baby. The baby died later that night with his mother holding him and with his dad telling him he was there. They gave him what he was trying to tell us he needed all along: his parents.

In God's Palm

~

Nancy Leigh Harless, ARNP

*"Courage doesn't always roar. Sometimes
it is that quiet voice at the end of the day
saying tomorrow I will begin again."*

—Anonymous

"WHY'D YOU GO and take your baby off the titty?"
Felicita demanded in a loud, lyrical voice. A dark scowl
wrinkled her broad, black forehead. "Now why'd ya go
and do that?"

Felicita, nurse for the surrounding villages, towered
before the group of tiny Mayan women who stood in the
middle of the road. An immense woman in both height
and girth, her blue striped seersucker uniform suggested
a military milieu. With both hands on her broad hips,
she looked vexed and frustrated and was such a formidable presence that I, along with every other woman in
the group, knew we were all in serious trouble.

Felicita allowed me, a North American nurse, to observe her immunization clinics in the villages that day. She was the public health nurse for Columbia Village and the dozen or so smaller villages in a 20-mile radius of her clinic. Columbia Village is in southern Belize, about 15 miles north of the Guatemala border.

Felicita's clinic was a dank, unpainted concrete block building in the center of Columbia Village. On the days when she wasn't traveling to the smaller surrounding village to do outreach and immunizations, her clinic was open for whatever medical emergency might appear. She treated everything from the exotic snakebite to the mundane bloody nose. She lived in a small apartment above her clinic and was on-call 24 hours a day. This is the norm for all rural nurses in Belize.

Nursing requires four years of university in Belize, the equivalent of a baccalaureate degree in the States. The training is intense and arduous, as well it must be since the rural public health nurse must function essentially as a complete health-care system for her entire area. Felicita wasn't simply the village nurse. The scope of her practice was awesome. She was the nurse, doctor, social worker, midwife, and ambulance service for her villages.

As we entered each village, Eltario, Felicita's driver, blasted the truck horn to alert the mothers we were coming. We stopped in the middle of the dusty road, climbed out of the truck, and lowered the tailgate to serve as an exam table. Candeleria, Felicita's assistant, climbed up in the back of the truck and slid two cardboard boxes forward to our reach. The village clinic was ready.

Within minutes, women in a rainbow of bright traditional dress emerged from their thatched-roof huts. Toddlers and older children trailed behind. The women carried their babies in white cotton slings across their backs, a supporting band across their foreheads. They each seemed to know their own part in the choreography of a village clinic. Felicita queried each mother about her own health, her baby's health, and then the rest of the family. At the same time, she drew up the immunizations.

One at a time the shy, gentle, browned-skinned women handed their baby-filled slings to me. Using the same block-and-tackle equipment used by fishermen to weigh fish, I held the apparatus up high and read aloud each baby's weight for Candeleria to record. Eltario wandered off to afford the women privacy.

Most of the mothers brought an empty jar or can for the liquid acetaminophen Felicita poured from a gallon jar. New mothers and any others who forgot were sent scampering back to their grass-thatched hut in search of a container for the cherry-red elixir.

"If the baby feels hot or is fussy, give him one spoonful in the morning and one at lunch and one in the evening," she told them. "If he feels hot in the night, give him one spoonful."

I wondered whether they even had spoons in their primitive little huts and, if so, what size? But the system here seemed to be working, so my questions were merely passing thoughts, flitting through my head like rain-forest butterflies without real need for an answer.

A worn-looking young woman stepped forward with her baby. Her tired face and the dullness in her dark eyes spoke volumes. I saw the weariness from struggling hard to live off the land, a deep-drained tired that ran clear to her core.

She handed me her baby-filled sling and softly announced, "Emitario." The sling was feather light. *This must be a newborn*, I thought. Then Candeleria pulled his card from the cardboard file and announced his birth date. Little Em was four months old! Holding the block and tackle high above my head, I looped his sling on the hook. A chill passed through me as I read his weight out loud—about eight pounds, not nearly enough for a four-month-old baby.

Felicita's broad brow wrinkled into a skeptical frown. She stepped closer, reread the scale, peered inside the baby-filled hammock, then turned toward the mother. She put both hands on her broad hips and asked bluntly, "Do you give your baby the titty?"

Looking away, the mother mumbled, "No, not anymore."

The tirade began. "Why'd ya take your baby off the titty? Now why'd ya go and do that?" Felicita thundered. "Don't you know there's nothing in the world better for him?"

"He stopped. He was sick almost a month ago with the diarrhea and he won't suck now," the young mother mumbled, looking at the ground.

Felicita came alive. Concern flashed in her dark eyes. "Does he still have diarrhea?" she asked, taking tiny Emitario, sling and all, from me.

"No, not now," the young mother replied defensively, sensing Felicita's disapproval. "He did for one week. He will suck the bottle, so I put honey in it for him to get him strong,"

Sitting on the tailgate of the truck, Felicita slowly removed tiny Emitario from his hammock and gently undressed him. Dry, loose skin hung on his frail, birdlike bones. His eyes were sunken and lacked the shine and sparkle of a healthy baby; they held only dull acceptance. He did not cry as she examined him, nor did he struggle away from her. It was as if this baby boy accepted he was no longer of this world.

Felicita barked orders to me to dig into a cardboard box and find the electrolyte solution mix. I rummaged deep but found only two packets, enough for two quarts. The baby was both dehydrated and malnourished. An ominous shadow passed over. I didn't know the statistics specifically for Belize, but I did know conservative estimates for all Third World countries say that every minute, eight babies die—mostly from infection, malnutrition, or diarrhea. *Two quarts will not make much difference*, I thought to myself.

"You must mix this powder with water and give to Em every hour until it is gone. Do you have sugar and salt in your home?" Felicita demanded.

"Yes," the woman whispered, looking at the ground.

Still, in a no-nonsense manner, she instructed the young mother to boil water and mix six spoons of sugar and four pinches of salt in the water. "Give it to him every hour until I come back. We must get special milk for Em until he learns to nurse again. For now, you tell your man he must get canned milk for your baby. Emitario is very, very sick. You must teach little Em how to suck again." In an encouraging voice, she continued, "With only a few weeks since he stopped, it may be possible."

Then, loudly, for the benefit of all the women gathered in the middle of the road, Felicita announced, "There is nothing in the world better for your babies than the milk from your titty. If the baby stops sucking, he will not grow. He will become sick. Honey is not good for your baby. It can make him sick. Titty is good for your baby. It will make your baby strong and thick."

I admired how she turned this tragedy into a learning experience for all the village women and felt a swell of respect for this pragmatic, plain-speaking nurse.

We completed the weights, exams, and immunizations and headed down the road, where we repeated the same process again and again in village after village until the day was spent. I, too, was spent. I felt bone-tired, weary, and so, so wretched. In three days Felicita would return to the village to assess little Emitario, but she told me that she wasn't optimistic.

"He is so little. She is so tired," she said.

We drove down the bumpy, dusty road in silence, reversing the early-morning route that brought us to the isolated villages. I offered to buy the formula for little Em, but Felicita looked sadly out of the truck window toward the horizon as she replied, "And can you buy the milk next week and next month and the next and the next and the next? No, buying milk will not help this baby or the other village babies." She turned toward me. Her sad but steady gaze met mine. Then, with a slight shrug, she looked away and softly sighed. "He's already in God's palm."

Such a challenging job! Such a formidable presence! Felicita is fearless. She plunges into her work every day and encourages women to take charge of their lives. She supports and applauds them to do their very best. Then, recognizing what she can't change, she accepts it all unconditionally. And every day when the sun drops below the towering rain-forest trees in the calm surrender of evening, Felicita knows that tomorrow she will begin again.

A New Life in My Charge

~

Karen Klein, RN

LIKE MOST NEW parents, when I first had my son, I was a bit overwhelmed by the feeling of responsibility that comes with having a newborn. Unlike most new parents, I am a nurse, so I easily adapted to the caregiver role.

The first night home from the hospital I remember thinking, "this is just like caring for a private-duty pediatric patient." The only thing was, the private-duty shift I was now starting for this particular pediatric patient would be 24 hours a day, 365 days a year, for the next 18 years! It certainly was intimidating, but again, I felt confident that I could do this and that my child would benefit from having a mother who is a nurse. I had worked for a few years in pediatric emergency rooms and knew what to expect from a neonate, so I was not overly worried about the little things that might trouble a new parent without such a background. Caring for the umbilical cord site, bathing, changing, holding, and feeding were all second nature. I was not alarmed by bad skin, multiple mustard-colored stools, or frequent sneezing and hiccups.

However, when my son began vomiting some of his feedings at two and a half weeks of age, I brought him to his pediatrician. She examined him and said it could be pyloric stenosis, a condition in some newborns whereby the muscle that controls food leaving the stomach to the small intestines is overdeveloped, preventing food from leaving the stomach. This causes the infant to vomit his feedings, with subsequent dehydration, and, without corrective surgery, eventual starvation and death.

I was horrified! How could my son have such a thing? Would my newborn have to undergo surgery? I put these thoughts out of my mind. Of course he would be just fine.

I was encouraged when the pediatrician gave him a trial feeding of glucose water in the office and he held it down. The doctor also told me she didn't feel the classic "olive" when palpating his abdomen, a common sign of pyloric stenosis, but she added that this usually occurs at three to six weeks of age, and my son was just two and a half weeks old. She sent me home with instructions to give the baby a half-and-half mixture of slightly warm chamomile tea and glucose water. If he kept it down, I should begin to feed him but give Pedialyte if he vomited anything after that, with the occasional bit of chamomile to settle the stomach. She said if he began projectile vomiting, or vomiting every feeding, then I should bring him back to the office or go to an emergency room.

Over the next few days, my baby did keep some of his feedings down and vomited others, usually after he was fed, burped, and laid in the crib, so I couldn't tell if it was projectile. I kept giving my "nursing care," trying to keep him hydrated. But four days later, when my son had a bilious odor to his breath and only two wet diapers, I brought him to the emergency room at the hospital, since it was Sunday morning and his doctor was not in the office.

The nurses were helpful and sympathetic, but the pediatric surgeon who was called to evaluate my son and start an intravenous chastised me that the baby was extremely dehydrated and I should have brought him in sooner. I felt terrible guilt. Obviously, I would never want any harm to come to my child. I told him that I was trying to keep up the fluids and hoped the vomiting would lessen, but the surgeon remained unsympathetic. Again I felt terrible and kept thinking, "Why didn't I seek medical attention a day or two sooner? A 'normal' parent probably would have run her kid to the ER after one day. I'm a bad nurse *and* a bad mother."

Later that day, after speaking with a few close friends, some of whom are nurses, I realized that part of me just couldn't accept that my perfect baby might need an operation, while another part was so used to dealing with very sick people that I was not as easily alarmed as a parent who wasn't a nurse might be. I supposed, too, that I thought since I was a skilled nurse, I could manage the illness. I concluded that being a nurse was not completely beneficial when it came to parenting. I should have recognized the adage well known by health care providers: When it comes to caring for a loved one, no medical professional, no matter how competent, can be completely objective.

The surgeon had said he felt the classic "olive" and the ultrasound had confirmed the diagnosis of pyloric stenosis. My baby would need a simple 20-minute operation to surgically split the muscle, which would relieve the obstruction, and then he'd be fine. He told me that my son would be put on the operating room schedule and later they'd let me know when the surgery would take place. Until then, the baby would be given intravenous fluids for hydration and be NPO (given nothing by mouth).

This alone was difficult, since it's natural for a baby to want to suckle. On Monday morning, when a resident informed me that my son would not be operated on until the next morning, I told him it was a shame that my baby couldn't feed for another day.

"It's okay, he won't get dehydrated since he's getting IV fluids," he told me.

"Tell *him* that," I responded, glancing at my baby. "He only knows he has a hungry belly."

For two days in total, I stood by and helplessly watched as my poor baby cried continually between sleep periods. I tried to comfort him by dipping a pacifier in glucose water and putting it in his mouth when he cried. He would suck a little but upon realizing there was no food, would spit out the pacifier and wail even louder. His tiny cheeks had developed a rash from rubbing the sheets and thrashing his head back and forth, crying for food that I could not provide. I cried too. I felt so powerless.

Also, the thought of the operation itself lurked unnervingly in the back of my mind. As a nurse, I was fully aware of all the possible complications that could occur, even with a "simple" operation. What if the anesthesiologist gave too much anesthesia and my son went into a permanent coma? Or he became hypoxic (lost oxygen to the brain) somehow during the operation and ended up with encephalopathy? Wouldn't it be terrible, I worried, if after nine months of concern about having a healthy baby and then the relief of having one, I ended up with a child who was permanently brain damaged at three weeks of age? This was my biggest fear—in many ways worse than death, which I presume would be the worst fear of a parent without a medical background. I told this to the surgeon and the anesthesiologist, who responded regarding the delivery of anesthesia, "Not too much, not too little, just the right amount, that's what we'll give him."

He was so confident but again, I felt so helpless. My vulnerable, six-pound-three-ounce newborn son's life was all in their hands. I had no choice in the matter; I had to depend on the skills of other medical professionals now. There was no part for me, the knowledgeable nurse, in this instance. Or was there?

The answer came a short time later, when two pediatric medical residents came into my son's hospital room and before I knew it, whisked my baby out to another examining room, which I could not locate, despite my best efforts. When they returned some 15 minutes later, they informed me that they'd done an arterial blood gas (a painful needle stick), a procedure they didn't like to do in front of the parent since it can be upsetting. That was unnecessary, I told them, because I was a nurse. But the resident responded, "No you're not. You're the patient's mother."

His words struck me: He was right. I wasn't the nurse; I was the mother. From that point on, I decided that when it came to this new life in my charge, I was a mother first, then a nurse. That was my role.

On Tuesday morning, the successful operation finally took place. While my 22-day-old son was in surgery, I reflected on this new life that had come into mine. I had felt the awesome responsibility and protectiveness imbued in parenthood just as most new parents do. But unlike most new parents, because of this experience I also realized that no matter how much I loved and cared for my child, there would be some things from which I could not shield him. Loving mother or capable nurse, I simply could not control some things in life. Most parents come to realize they can't protect their child from every painful life experience when the child is older—school age or a teen. But I learned this unfortunate reality when my son was still very new to life.

Today my son is a happy, healthy 18-year-old college student. He has never had any complications from the pyloric stenosis, though from the corrective surgery he does have a one-inch scar in the middle of his abdomen.

Over the years, every time I've seen this scar it has reminded me that where he is concerned, I'm a mother first, then a nurse.

As well, it always reminds me that, unfortunately, I can't protect him from every difficult, painful experience in life. I can only help him to deal with all of life's experiences—the good and the bad.

My Story

~

Monica Frommer, RN

Eɪɢʜᴛ ʏᴇᴀʀꜱ ᴀɢᴏ, I delivered my first daughter at
Cedars Sinai Medical Center. My husband and I had the
most incredible labor and delivery experience, all thanks
to a registered nurse who stayed at my bedside throughout
my entire 11 hours of labor and delivery. This particular
evening was unusually slow for the hospital and I was the
only patient my nurse had to care for. She was at our bedside until my daughter was delivered and resting safely on
my chest. This nurse was kind, patient, compassionate,
knowledgeable, and genuine. She seemed to bask in the
happiness of people who surrounded her.

As I watched her, it suddenly dawned on me that she
held the position of my dreams, a nurse who actually got
paid to participate in the world's most miraculous event:
childbirth.

My husband and I were scared, and I remember how nice it was to be guided step by step through this overwhelming time. She explained everything that was happening to our baby as well as to me, greatly reducing our anxiety. Once the baby was back in the room with us, the nurse helped my husband hold her properly. She helped me nurse my daughter for the first time. Even after spending all the tiring hours of my labor with us, she did not simply dump us off on the next nurse; although her shift was ending, she continued to take an extra few minutes to explain where we were going to be moved to next, and what to expect with the baby in the upcoming hours of our hospital stay.

The time came for us to say good-bye to our wonderful nurse. We were moved to a regular postpartum recovery room, where we were introduced to our new nurse. This is when things started to go wrong. We were oriented to the room, and the nurse checked my blood pressure and made sure my bleeding was under control, as well as our baby's breathing, heart rate, and temperature. From that point on we hardly saw her again. We were introduced to two more nurses, who through our short hospital stay also seemed to be stressed and short for time. We felt as though we burdened the nurses whenever we asked them for anything. Although we were in a hospital, we soon learned we were pretty much on our own. The nurses were nice and apologized for their lack of time; however, they had to deal with an overwhelming load of paperwork and more critical patients, such as those who had delivered via cesarean section, or the patients who simply used their call light a little too much, leaving us feeling alone and scared with many questions left unanswered about our new baby.

About 24 hours later, another new nurse came in to tell us it was time to go home. I looked at my husband's pale, scared face. We had no idea what to expect and wondered if we would be able to take care of this innocent baby all by ourselves. We wished we could have someone help us at home. I did have my mother, who came and helped here and there, but mostly we were on our own. I remember wondering how something as natural as breast-feeding a baby could feel so awkward. I felt incompetent and tired, was sleep deprived, and felt like I needed some special attention for myself.

Luckily, little by little, I did end up getting the hang of things. I was an at-home mom for a while. Shortly after celebrating my daughter's first birthday, I decided that I would pursue the postpartum nursing field. I knew I wanted to work with women and their newborn babies, giving them all the time and care that my labor and delivery nurse gave to me. I took classes and finished college, becoming a licensed vocational nurse. I immediately went to work in the labor and delivery unit in Northridge Hospital, where they had me cross-trained to work in the newborn care nursery and postpartum care, as well as to be an emergency C-section technician. I continued to take classes and entered the Registered Nursing Ladder program. I completed my rotations in Cedars Sinai Hospital working in the pediatric, newborn nursery, and postpartum care units.

Upon earning my registered nurse license it dawned on me that no matter what hospital I ended up working at, the hospital bureaucracy and constant chaos would always stand in the way of doing the kind of nursing I always knew deep down inside I wanted to provide. A mountain of paperwork and the high number of patients assigned to me made me feel like the quality of care I was providing was way below my standards. I never went home at the end of the day feeling the way I had hoped I would. I wanted to make sure that my patients wouldn't go home scared and clueless, the way I had been sent home with my daughter.

I began to look into different types of nursing positions and found home health care to be the most promising. After practicing pediatric home health care for only six weeks, I immediately knew I had found my passion. I knew there was no way I would ever work in a hospital again. One-on-one care, guidance, and instruction was suddenly a reality.

The relationships I develop with my clients are difficult to describe in words. Not only do I have the opportunity to get paid to do what I love, but when I leave my clients' homes, I don't feel as though my work is done, I feel as though I have made lifetime friends.

Currently I work with a registry per diem in the pediatric division and have my own business caring for private clients as a postpartum registered nurse. I have a wonderful, supportive husband of over eight years, and last but certainly not least, I am a proud mother of two daughters ages eight and six, and a three-year-old son.

Changing Assignments

~

Nicole M. Jarrell, MSN, RNC

MY LOVE FOR neonatal nursing developed during a nurse externship program in the neonatal intensive care unit at the hospital affiliated with the university I was attending. I learned early on that becoming a neonatal nurse would bring both joy and heartache. But to me, the joy I received from the successes we celebrated in caring for these fragile infants far outweighed the occasional heartaches. I felt it was my calling in life.

After a very rewarding career for ten years as a neonatal nurse, I decided to broaden my scope of practice. I had always been intrigued with neonatal cardiac surgery and upon relocating, had an opportunity to work in a pediatric cardiac intensive care unit. Working in the CICU, I would still be able to utilize my neonatal expertise, since approximately half of the patients were neonates, but

I would be challenged with learning the pediatric population as well. Often as a neonatal nurse, I wondered what happened to those infants later on in their lives. Neonatal cardiac surgery would give me the opportunity to experience following these babies across the continuum, something not possible in the NICU.

I made the transition well and developed expertise in neonatal and pediatric cardiac nursing. I quickly learned that CICU nursing has the same joys and heartaches that occur in the NICU. Although I was able to care for patients of many different ages, I still was drawn to my original calling and the neonates were always my favorite patients. This story is about a very special CICU baby and his family.

I glanced across the desk as I was waiting to receive report on my two patients for the day and noticed my friend was frowning. I asked her what was wrong, and she explained that she was assigned to take a patient from the operating room instead of my two patients whom she had cared for the day before. The charge nurse had thought that she was giving her a break, but she really wanted her original two patients instead, so I offered to change assignments and admit the patient from the operating room. After making the offer, I hesitated and laughed, saying to her, "I should have asked what the patient is having done first!" I learned that the baby was having a Blalock-Taussig (BT) shunt placed. This normally is a relatively uncomplicated surgery with a quick recovery and short hospitalization, so I thought it was a great trade. Little did I realize at the time what an impact that change would have.

Baby Alex was already in the operating room, so I spent the morning preparing for the day's surgical patients and helping other staff. Time went on, and still no baby. There were unexpected complications in the OR. When Alex finally was brought to the unit after the operation, he was extremely unstable. He had a severe capillary leak and had developed ascites and pleural effusions. The surgeon had placed multiple chest tubes and a peritoneal Jackson-Pratt (JP) drain in order to evacuate the fluid. Alex was losing fluid through these drains faster than I could replace it with fresh-frozen plasma into his circulation, and he was in hypovolemic shock. This was an ominous sign. The charge nurse came by to check on the baby and said to me, "He's going to die." I replied, "I know, I don't want to hear it!" Only one other time in over 15 years of nursing practice had I seen a patient with capillary leak this severe survive. I hoped and prayed that Alex would be the second.

His family came to his bedside aware that there were complications from the surgery, but unaware of how drastically his prognosis had changed. The surgeon's approach was to take it "one day at a time," and he refused to acknowledge even to himself that this baby might not survive. Alex's parents, Ann* and Mark,* were wonderful, and that made this already difficult situation even more heartbreaking.

Ann's pregnancy happened shortly after Mark's grandfather's death. It was both unexpected and high risk, due to her advanced maternal age. After recovering from the initial shock, Ann and Mark were elated about the upcoming addition to their current family of four, which included their 16-year-old daughter and Ann's adult son from her first marriage. The anticipation of Alex's arrival brought joy and hope back to a family that was going through grief and despair. The family was blissfully unaware of the peril that Alex was in.

Alex's heart defect was found during a routine ultra-sound in the second trimester of Ann's pregnancy. Ann's obstetrician referred her to a pediatric cardiologist for a fetal echo and prenatal consultation. She shared with me that all she had comprehended from that meeting was that during Alex's first week of life, he would have the first of the three surgeries required to "fix" his heart. Afterward, he would be in the hospital for ten days and then would need close follow-up care from his local cardiologist. She never had grasped the gravity of his heart defect, pulmonary atresia with intact septum and sinusoids. Ann and Mark realized that Alex wasn't recovering as quickly as expected when post-op day number ten came and went with Alex still on the ventilator and in critical condition. However, they still were oblivious to the gravity of the situation and Alex's true prognosis. Since it is not the role of the nurse to share that information, I was constantly torn with that knowledge and the need to provide hope and support to Ann and Mark.

Alex's constant capillary leak, ascites, and pleural effusions made it impossible to successfully wean him from the ventilator. His nutritional status was affected by his inability to tolerate feedings, thus necessitating continued supplementation with hyperalimentation. His liver was impacted both from the hyperalimentation and venous congestion. He was beginning to have multisystem organ failure, and Mark was putting the pieces together. It had been about three weeks since Alex's surgery when Mark confronted me. Ann had gone to the Ronald McDonald house to shower and rest, leaving Mark alone at Alex's bedside. He questioned me regarding Alex's prognosis and forced me to tell the truth. He said that he was tired of the physicians beating around the bush and not being totally honest with him and Ann. They had asked the surgeon daily what he thought, and his response was always "I'm hopeful that he will recover" or "I'm not ready to give up yet; we just need to have patience." I could not lie to Mark, so I answered his questions honestly.

Right or wrong, when our patients in the CICU have a strong nurse who has developed a good rapport with a family, our physicians often leave it up to the nurse to answer those tough questions. When the physicians have those difficult conversations with the family, it is often the nurses who answer the onslaught of questions that come after the initial shock is gone. Sometimes it is a matter of trust. The physicians come and go, but it is the nurse that spends 12 hours at the bedside day after day with the child and his or her family. Primary nursing plays such an important role in the care and support of these critical patients and families. I was Alex's day-shift primary nurse and therefore played an important role in coordinating his plan of care and naturally, supporting his parents. Alex also had both night- and weekend-shift primaries. It was rare that he would have a "non-primary" nurse assigned because he had such a diverse team of primaries providing his care.

So what did I tell Mark that day? My answers to his questions were straightforward. When he asked me directly whether Alex was going to make it home, my reply was, "Not without a miracle. But, I believe in miracles and I have seen them happen." I described what improvements needed to happen in order for Alex to survive and explained that if those things did not start to happen, his body's organs would continue to fail. Upon Ann's return, Mark gently broke the news to her. Ann wanted to know how much longer Alex could hang on and when would it be best for them to stop his care if he was going to die. I explained that at this point in time, we were all still holding onto hope because his body was not yet beyond the capability of recovery, even though the chances were slim. When all hope is gone, then it would be time to stop, and we would let them know as that time approached. I also encouraged them to keep their communication open and honest with each other. They needed to agree upon all of the decisions that they would have to make in the upcoming days so that later on, they would not second-guess themselves. They had to know and believe in their minds and hearts that they had been good parents and had made the best choices for their son. They would have to live with these choices for the rest of their lives. Ann and Mark had shared with me about their strong faith in God and that they didn't want to give up. However, Ann was fearful about how Alex's death would occur and was adamant that she wanted to be holding him when he died. I explained that it is sometimes predictable, but that other times the heart just stops without warning. Knowing their faith basis, I explained that only God knew of what was to come and that how Alex's death occurred would be what was best for their family. I encouraged them to hold onto their hope and faith until they felt peace that it was time to let go. I continued to reassure and support them over the days following to reaffirm their choice to continue his care and then ultimately choose the time to let go.

The day he died was both eventful and peaceful, just the way Mark and Ann wanted it to be. Many family members and friends came to comfort them, some completely unaware of the situation before their arrival at the hospital. Ann said that having so many visitors and everyone having a chance to see Alex before his death was important to her and was exactly what she needed. All of Alex's primary nurses were in frequent contact, and some came both to provide their support and to say their goodbyes to Alex, Ann, and Mark. I was on duty and was his assigned nurse for the day.

That afternoon, Ann and Mark made the decision that they were ready to withdraw Alex's support to allow him to die peacefully. Per the hospital's policy, Alex's surgeon was his primary physician and would have to agree with their decision, along with two other attending physicians. Historically, the surgeons are often the last of the team to be ready to accept death, so sometimes the families request to change to the cardiologist, removing the surgeon from responsibility for their child's care. Cardiologists often have a more realistic and holistic approach and are more accepting and supportive of families' decisions. The attending cardiologist knew the surgeon was going to have difficulty with this decision, so she discussed with him Ann and Mark's wishes prior to his arrival at Alex's bedside. She gently reminded him that this was their baby, not his, and that it was medically appropriate to withdraw support; therefore the decision was really theirs to make, and he needed to put his personal feelings aside and support the parents. Reluctantly, he relented and respected their wishes.

Alex's family members all came in and several took the opportunity to hold him; for most, it was both a first and last time. When they were ready, we stopped his cardiac medication drips and extubated him. Ann rocked him as he died peacefully, surrounded by his loving family. Ann and Mark stayed with him to assist in his care as they had done so many times before. Mark gave him one last massage, this time with no wires or tubes in the way. It was a touching experience and I was privileged to participate. We finished his care, packed his belongings, and the time to leave was approaching. I sensed that Ann, who was holding him, could not bear to put him back into his bed. Instead, I asked her to hand him to me so that her last memory of him would not be in the bed, but rather being held and loved.

I have followed up with Ann and Mark since Alex's death, both as a part of the bereavement program and as a friend. Ann shared with me one of the most important lessons that I have learned as a nurse. She said the most important thing I ever said to her was that only God knew of what was to come and that whatever was best for their family was what would happen...it was not in our control. Often as nurses we try hard to retain control, but it is a battle we cannot win. She said that she held onto that statement and that was exactly how it happened. She said that if she had tried to plan for that final day, she could not have imagined anything better than what occurred. She said that even though it was the hardest thing she has ever done, she knew beyond a shadow of a doubt that they made the right decision and Alex's death happened exactly according to God's plan to meet their needs...even down to their nurse being changed on the day of his operation.

Icarus Again

~

Julianna Paradisi, RN

THE TRANSPORT CALL came at 5 A.M. and the assignment was mine. The transferring hospital was a 15-minute
flight from Portland. We would depart and return to our
hospital's helipad, a scoop and run. My 12-hour nightshift
ended at 0730. Maybe I'd be back by then.

A pediatric intensive care nurse for six years, I trans-
ported patients occasionally. This was the last transport
of my career. Recognizing flight nursing had become
a specialty, our hospital had formed a dedicated transport team, but they would not activate for another week.
These nurses learned intubation, the insertion of umbilical lines and chest tubes. They mixed drips. They wore
flight suits.

While packing equipment for this transport, I
remembered my training. The pilot showed me a locator

box in the tail of the helicopter. If we crashed, I would have to get to the box and push a button that released a radio transmission, signaling rescuers to the crash location. I laughed, imagining myself wearing green scrubs, a hospital-supplied, poly-fill parka, and white Nikes, crashing in the middle of the night into the snow on top of Mt. Hood, and my unlikely survival of the event to use the locator and await rescue. I preferred working at the bedside, with my feet on the ground. I had not applied for a position with the new transport team.

Our patient was a 10-day-old newborn at a small hospital in Oregon. The transferring physician had called our pediatric ICU intensivist and reported a bacterial infection. The newborn was stable, so the intensivist elected not to accompany the transport team. Instead, he would meet us in the unit when we returned. This is a common practice in hospitals. A flight nurse and a respiratory therapist accompanied me. The flight nurse, highly skilled in adult trauma, knew the flight protocol and was our liaison with the pilot. He lacked experience in neonatal and pediatric nursing, but that was my area of expertise. We didn't expect any problems.

Here's the problem with transports: The patient's reported condition is relative to the expertise and clinical experience of the transferring physician. No physician can be a clinical expert in every aspect of medicine. Instead, specialists working in tertiary care facilities provide expert care. Pediatrics is a specialty few small hospitals maintain and in which only large facilities specialize. The parents had taken this baby to a pediatrician two days earlier, reporting flu-like symptoms. The pediatrician prescribed antibiotics, but their baby's symptoms worsened, so they brought him to this emergency room. The doctor recognized they had a sick newborn on their hands and rightly assessed that the baby needed the care of a specialized children's hospital. It seemed the baby had an infection, and that is what he reported.

Our team reached the hospital and unloaded the transport sled, IV pumps, and black medical bag containing a limited assortment of medications and supplies. I carried a cell phone to communicate with the intensivist in Portland. An emergency department nurse handed me the medical record, including a chest X-ray, in a manila envelope, saying the parents had already left for Portland in order to meet us at our hospital. I read the record and film. That was the last I saw of the transferring hospital's medical team. This is not unusual. On most transports that I've been on, once the transport team arrives and receives report, the transferring staff sign off and continue their work. They left, and it was just the four of us in a separate part of the emergency department.

The respiratory therapist made her way to the baby, already intubated and assisted with his breathing by a ventilator. The flight nurse put the IV tubes into our pumps, preparing for departure.

I looked at the monitors to write down vital signs before we loaded the neonate into the transport sled, placing both it and the portable ventilator into the helicopter. This is a "scoop and run," meaning that we simply wanted to get the baby and ourselves back to the PICU, where the intensivist and day-shift nurses could take over. Looking at the patient, I realized it was not going to happen this time.

My attention focused on the baby's face. Intubated, he could not cry, but his tightly squinted eyes and grimace shouted, "I'm dying, help me!" It is an expression I've seen before on adults experiencing severe chest pain. It expresses their feeling of impending doom. I thought, "He's having a heart attack." I can still picture his tiny face.

Scanning the monitor, my own heart sank as I saw that the ventilator was delivering 100 percent oxygen through the breathing tube, but his oxygen saturations were very low, and dropping. The numbers I read on the monitor indicated that he was not getting enough oxygen in his bloodstream to sustain life, and we were already giving him as much as possible through the ventilator. His heart rate and blood pressure were normal, but that wasn't going to last very long if we didn't correct the oxygenation problem. I remembered to breathe, and asked the RT if the ventilator was connected to oxygen and working properly. It was; she had already checked. The vent delivered what should have been an effective respiratory rate. The RT took the baby off the vent and began hand-bagging while I suctioned the tube. I pulled out the chest X-ray from the envelope, looking at it again to reconfirm the endotracheal tube was in the right place. It was. The lungs were clear. There were no secretions when we suctioned. This was surprising in an infant suspected to have a bacterial infection. The heart, however, looked enlarged.

Using the cell phone, a big, boxy behemoth from the 1990s, I called our intensivist to report my findings, anxious for him to tell me what to do next. As in many old hospital buildings, the walls of the room may have been lined with lead, because I couldn't get the call through, so I went to an adjacent hallway to make that call and every other call during this episode. I could not see my patient or read the monitor from the hallway. The call dropped and I had to redial. Irritation compounded my rising fear. Finally, the call went through. Words rushed out as I gave report, and my anxiety manifested through the phone. Expecting to hear we were on our way back, the intensivist was caught off guard.

"Check the X-ray," he said, "is the tube is in the right place?"

"I've done that, the lungs are clear, the tube's okay," I repeated.

"Well, reposition the tube and get a blood gas," was the order.

The RT helped me reposition the tube while the flight nurse looked for someone to take the blood test to the lab for processing. The repositioned tube did not help, and the test results confirmed that our patient was in respiratory failure and worsening. The pulses in the baby's feet and wrists were faint. Then his heart rate and blood pressure began dropping, signs of impending cardiac arrest, and a full code. I was scared. Returning to the hallway, I got the intensivist back on the phone. By this time, I was convinced that we were not dealing with a bacterial infection, and I told him so.

"This isn't sepsis; I think its cardiogenic shock. I want to start PGE1." PGE1 is a medication administered as a continuous IV drip and causes the ductus arteriosus to open. The ductus arteriosus, a tiny door between the main pulmonary artery and the aorta, allows circulation of oxygenated blood in the fetus while it's attached by the umbilical cord to the placenta. After the baby is born and able to breathe air, this opening usually closes in the first week or so of life. In this case, I knew that it had already begun closing. I wanted it to stay open, because oxygenated blood from the lungs would flow into the parts of his heart that did not have it; at least that's what I hoped.

To summarize the situation, a highly skilled pediatric intensivist is in a hospital talking to a badly frightened nurse in another hospital, a several hours' drive away, at a time of day when most people are asleep. The intensivist was told by another doctor that the patient has a bacterial infection, is stable, and is ready to transport. This nurse, who has been up all night, is so anxious that she is talking too fast. She cannot see the patient or monitor when she is on the phone, so she is running back and forth from room to room in order to answer the intensivist's questions about the patient. Sometimes the call is dropped. He cannot see any of this, and wonders, "What's going on?" The nurse tells him that the emergency room doctor is wrong, it's a heart defect, not an infection, and the baby is dying. Moreover, this nurse is telling him what medication she wants to give.

The intensivist had the responsibility to question my assessment. He had to decide between my assessment and that of another doctor. Could he trust me? I was pretty damn sure I was right. He told me, "Start PGE1 and get back here!" I asked how fast to start the infusion. "Just start it and get back!" He practically yelled. He wanted us back, so he could see for himself. I believed the baby could not survive the trip. I wanted him to have a chance. The helicopter is a very small place, mostly dark. Our team's radio contact with one another and the intensivist would be limited. Performing a full code in the helicopter while in flight was nearly impossible. The baby wasn't stable enough to survive even that short journey.

I needed a rate for the PGE1. I called the PICU and talked to the charge nurse. I asked her to calculate the rate for me. Medication doses and IV rates for children are based on their weights, and each dose is calculated individually for every patient. The PICU had preprinted rate sheets for PGE1.

As we spoke, a pediatric cardiologist walked into the PICU. Overhearing our conversation, he realized I was on transport. "What's she got?" he asked. She told him. He said, "She's got a left hypoplast. Tell her to run it at this rate." "Cardiology says it's a hypoplastic left," she told me, "and here's your order for the PGE1."

I exhaled. I was no longer afraid that my assessment was wrong. We started the PGE1 and administered some fluids. The newborn's blood pressure increased, and he stabilized. I thought we could get back with him alive— not well, but alive. Seizing the opportunity, we grabbed our equipment and loaded the sled. I didn't take my eyes off the monitor. Nearing Portland, the flight nurse informed me via the radio transmitter in our helmets that we'd do a "hot load" once we hit the helipad, meaning we would disembark the helicopter and unload the patient while the rotor blades were turning. "Keep your head down," he admonished.

We left the pad safely and entered the hospital. The baby's blood pressure dropped again, dangerously low. Reaching the PICU on the fifth floor, we ran through its double automatic doors past a gauntlet of doctors and staff waiting for our arrival. News of the baby's deteriorating condition had traveled throughout the Children's Hospital. Gowned and gloved, our intensivist was ready to place central lines into the patient. The cardiologist stood silently behind him and we made eye contact. Someone asked me if I knew where surgical caps were stored. "Fuck caps" was the last thing I remember saying, "I need a dopamine drip STAT."

I charted this Transport from Hell in the nurse's notes, drove home, and went to bed. I had the next three days off, during which I relived the entire transport over and over again in my head, questioning everything I'd done and said, angry for being in that situation and worrying whether I had made the baby's condition worse. At times, I considered calling the PICU and finding out what had happened, but quite frankly, I was afraid I would hear that I had made a horrible mistake and the baby had suffered for it. It was a long three days.

I would like to write that when I went back to work, the doctors had worked magic and the little baby was going to be just fine. I would like to write that I was a hero and that my recognition of his diagnosis and response to it saved his life. I was told that, indeed, the baby had been born with hypoplastic left heart syndrome, which is characterized by a nonexistent left ventricle or one too small to pump oxygenated blood effectively to the vital organs of the body. His heart, lungs, and kidneys were irreversibly damaged. He needed all three organs transplanted to survive with a chronically ill, and short, life span. Even if all of the organs were available in time, his chance of surviving such complex surgeries in his weakened state was unlikely. His heartbroken parents chose to let nature take its course, and he died in their arms in the PICU.

The futility of all I had done struck me like ice water thrown in my face. The baby had been doomed from birth.

The following week, transports at our hospital changed, improving the experience for everyone.

Over time, I've gleaned a small amount of peace knowing that the baby's parents were able to hold him again while he was still alive. He did not die in the night sky of Oregon, a rare Icarus in a haywire Greek myth. And I learned what I think most nurses and doctors know: We are human. We cannot always soar, as if we are gods.

The Cath Lab Baby

~

Vera Knox, RNC

I SUPPOSE I WAS always the kind of nurse that loved adrenaline rushes. Many people don't understand that it's not that loving nurses like bad things to happen so they can have their excitement fix, it's about making a difference.

One Memorial Day a few years back, two of our nurses were sent to the emergency room to monitor the unborn baby of a woman having a heart attack. I was intrigued by the situation and sad I had not been selected. But strangely, after a while the two registered nurses were called back to obstetrics, and I was sent to attend to the patient instead.

Once in the ER, I was shocked to see a woman (who I will call Virginia) in such agony. Of course, we deal with suffering women in obstetrics daily, but this was different.

I had never seen a person experiencing an acute heart attack. Knowing Virginia was pregnant, I felt a sudden discomfort with my responsibility, as I really knew absolutely nothing about caring for a patient like her. The ER nurses reassured me that all I had to do was make sure to monitor the unborn baby.

I watched the fetal monitor and was amazed at the strength of the unborn. It was running a normal fetal heart rate in the 120s, with no signs of distress. After the narcotics the mom had received, the baby seemed peacefully asleep in utero. Looking at the mom, I thought she looked "weathered," as if she had had a hard life. Soon I found out that she was only 39, and that she had been a cocaine addict who damaged her organs with the drug. My heart went out to her, and I hoped she would make the turn and become a good mom, if she survived.

An ER nurse came in and I asked whether the obstetrician had been notified. Yes, he had. But he had made a statement that this was a cardiac and not an obstetrical problem. I disagreed wholeheartedly.

A cardiologist visited Virginia—quite an unfriendly guy. I felt I had the right to participate in the plan and asked whether the patient might be approved to have a cesarean section today for the safety of the baby. Virginia was much too unstable to undergo surgery, he said. She also had had lots of heparin and could bleed to death. The plan was to go to the cath lab and search for the cause of the problem, then send her to the intensive care unit and have her stabilize for a couple of days. The baby could be delivered by C-section once this was achieved, if so advised by the obstetrician. The unborn baby was premature, but most likely better off in the outside world than inside such a sick mother, just not quite yet. The cardiologist made clear that he expected me to ensure fetal well-being at all times and to stay with the patient wherever she went.

In the meantime, I reported to my charge nurse. I wondered about her judgment. She wanted me to come back to OB when the patient was transferred to the ICU, as she could not spare a nurse for an entire shift sitting with one patient. I was told that after the transfer, I should go and check on the baby every couple of hours. What, to perhaps find the baby dead? ICU nurses don't know how to read a fetal monitor strip, just as I don't know how to read an EKG. I decided I would take this issue up with the house supervisor when the time came.

We transferred the patient to the cath lab. After many years employed at this hospital, I had never been there before. Since it was a holiday, the staffing seemed inadequate to me, but then I don't know how it usually is. There was the cardiologist, one registered nurse, a tech, and me.

The procedure was started with the patient awake. I tried to reassure her. Monitoring the baby during the procedure was easy, thank goodness, as the baby was already around 33 weeks. I watched and tried to understand what I was seeing on the screen. It was interesting to be part of this, but also scary. I felt a sudden insecurity. What if something happened? I was the only person in the room that knew anything about obstetrics, and what could I do by myself if things went wrong?

I don't remember the exact chain of events. At one point the cardiologist became very agitated and called for his partner. There was a major problem; I think a large vessel was almost completely occluded. It was decided to perform an emergency angioplasty. Things became hectic and I felt impending disaster. The second cardiologist arrived and the procedure was started.

Shortly thereafter, the patient was suddenly defibrillated. I had seen this only on ER shows. Virginia's body jumped off the table and I was afraid she might actually fall off. Amazingly, I saw no distress in the baby, only a brief disconnection of the heart rate tracing, and then it continued steadily into the 120s.

At this point I really needed support. I called my charge nurse and told her to call the obstetrician in *now*, briefly describing the current events. I couldn't believe the response: "That's not my job, have the cardiologist call him." Was she out of her mind? The cardiologist was trying to save the patient's life and he was in the middle of a sterile procedure.

I hung up the phone and paged the obstetrician myself. While I awaited his return phone call, the patient again was defibrillated, and again, the baby hung in there.

It seemed like an eternity before I was able to speak to the obstetrician. In the meantime Virginia's blood pressure was dropping severely, and I informed the nurse that the baby would not tolerate this kind of hypotension for long. The dopamine drip was immediately increased.

However, it didn't help. The blood pressure continued to drop, and suddenly my baby gave out. The heart rate dropped from 120 to 40 abruptly and never recovered.

In a way, I felt idiotic telling two cardiologists that an emergency C-section needed to be performed now. "Do something," I heard one say. It was completely out of their comfort zone. Out of mine, too.

What could I do? The obstetrician wasn't here yet; a nurse midwife wouldn't be able to perform surgery, so who could? I called the OB secretary, an awesome woman, and asked her to call the Kaiser obstetrician (and only candidate to be able to help) to the cath lab "stat." And to mobilize the entire OB staff to bring me everything I needed for a baby resuscitation—crash cart, warmer, transporter. Then I called a "Code Pink to the Cath Lab," meaning a baby resuscitation is necessary. We do this some time in advance when a baby is dying in utero and we expect a full code. That way, when the baby is delivered, all necessary support staff is at the bedside and ready.

An incredible turmoil started within the hospital. Staff was flying down hallways with equipment. Doctors and others got lost, because most OB staff really had no idea where the cath lab was. "By the Mickey Mouse," some were told. The giant Mickey Mouse in the hallway on the fourth floor was known to most, and quickly help arrived.

The Kaiser obstetrician, an extremely difficult man, arrived very soon. Usually he fussed about everything and was incredibly intimidating, so I was amazed at how he responded—completely focused on the task at hand. He didn't know the patient, trusted me that the baby was in severe trouble, told me calmly that he needed an OR crew, an OR setup, an anesthesia setup, and an anesthesiologist.

I called the OR and reinforced the severity of the emergency, and all that I needed. The teamwork was incredible, and all staff members we needed in the cath lab at this time were available. Within minutes everyone was there. But the anesthesiologist was afraid to give the patient a general anesthetic. Would she not survive it? I don't know. I do know that the Kaiser obstetrician was ready to cut Virginia with a local anesthetic. At this time the anesthesiologist reconsidered and a light general anesthesia was given. The C-section was started, the doctor proceeding rapidly, with no concern over sterility, just trying to save the little life. At this time I lost the baby's heart rate.

The obstetrician really had no time to think about which life to save, the mother's or baby's. Perhaps that was good. To perform such a major operation on Virginia in her state could cost her her life; not doing it surely would cost the baby's. The doctor did the best he could in trying to save both. I was very impressed.

Seventeen minutes after the heart rate first dropped to the 40s, the baby (I will call him Trevor) was born. The limp, blue body was handed to the team. They were ready, and the resuscitation went well. Everybody was amazed how good the initial outcome was, but I think we all wondered what the long-term status would be. I kept thinking about the six-minute period after which a brain is often damaged when not getting sufficient oxygenation.

Trevor was taken to our NICU, where he stayed for a while. Virginia went to the ICU and had a difficult recovery. One complication was that indeed, she bled internally and a large amount of blood had to be surgically evacuated later. Besides, she had severe heart problems and her kidneys seemed to be failing.

I was able to visit Virginia in the ICU a couple of times. She was gravely ill and needed a heart transplant, but she wasn't a candidate for the waiting list, due to her prior history. Fair, but sad.

Trevor went home with Virginia's sister. And when Virginia was discharged she moved into her sister's little home in Escondido. I visited her once, about six months after the heart attack. My curiosity about how she and Trevor were doing was overwhelming.

She occupied a small room in the house, with a tiny kitchen. It was very clean and tidy. On the floor sat a drooling, smiley-faced boy. I couldn't believe it. I handed him the stuffed puppy with long, floppy ears I had brought, and he instantly started chewing on its ear. There seemed to be absolutely no deficit. Trevor's father wasn't involved, but I could see by the little boy's eyes that his father must be Asian.

Virginia was delighted that I came to visit her. She told me she would love to hear what happened that day, as her sister kept all this a secret. Why, she didn't know. I had no reason not to tell her. So I explained everything I remembered that happened in the ER and cath lab on that Memorial Day, the way I'd experienced it.

During our talk, I noticed that Virginia was articulate but often lost her train of thought. Her attention span was short also. She apologized and stated she had retained some permanent problems after the event.

After I described how I perceived what happened in the cath lab that day, I asked Virginia to describe *her* experience.

She remembered having gone through "the tunnel" twice. The first time, she came to a stream and beyond it was a beautiful meadow. She saw her (deceased) mom in the meadow and wanted to cross the stream to join her. But her mom told her she needed to go back, and so she did.

The second time she came to the meadow, she actually stepped into the water. Her mom became very upset and told her that she had been irresponsible all her life, that her baby already didn't have a dad, and that she needed to be a good mom for him. She would have to return and take care of him. And so she did once more.

Virginia continued to struggle for her life in the ICU, while her son did very well. For days after the incident, I had thought that this woman must have had an angel watching over her, who helped save her son's and her life. When she told me that the entire time she was in ICU, an angel was sitting on her bed, I felt chills.

During the years to follow, I often thought of Virginia and Trevor. Occasionally I called them. When Trevor was about three, she told me that "Flapjack," the long-eared puppy, was his favorite toy. When he was five, she had moved into her own apartment. It made me happy to see her be independent. But her health was very poor and shortly after that, she passed away from a massive heart attack.

I can only say that having helped save the life of the "cath lab baby" was the highlight of my career. It makes me happy to know that Virginia and Trevor had time to get to know each other, and I hope at the time of her death he was old enough to retain some beautiful memories of his loving mother.

PART SIX

Nurses Who Challenge

Emily

~

Patricia Harman, RN, CNM, MSN

"COME ON, AMBER, you can do it," I entreated the
tired mother. Amber was a 28-year-old social worker whose
infant's head had been on the perineum for 45 minutes. I
glanced out the birthing-room window to see the predawn
light, a rim of silver under dark clouds.

Amber had been committed to going natural. She
had read all the books, gone to childbirth classes with her
husband, Darrell, and even practiced self-hypnosis. I'd
stayed up all night to help her. Now, just before the tape at
the end of the marathon, she'd run out of steam.

The young woman squatted on the bed, her eyes
closed, leaning her chin on the birthing bar. Her smooth,
round belly showed through her thin, blue hospital gown.
I frowned at the size of the bulge. *Maybe the baby is just
too big.*

Darrell caught my eye and stared without blinking. I knew what he was asking. Could his wife do this? Was there something wrong? Neither of us wanted to say anything discouraging, but in fact we were all losing steam.

"Amber, I know you're tired. We all are. Why don't you rest through the next few contractions? If the urge to push is too strong, just bear down a little. I want to call Dr. Harman. Maybe he can come in and help us." Dr. Harman is my husband and partner, my medical backup.

The registered nurse, Nancy, and I lowered the bed and eased our patient down on her side. I nodded to Darrell. In the carpeted hallway, outside the birthing room, I explained, "I know Amber wanted to have a natural birth and she's done great, but she's getting too tired to finish the job and the Pitocin isn't helping. When Dr. Harman comes, I think we should have him pull the baby out with a vacuum extractor. If we wait much longer she won't have the strength to help... It will still be a vaginal birth..."

Darrell nodded and brushed his long brown hair off his face. I could see the tears in his eyes, just floating on the rim. I patted him on his thin shoulder and went down the hall to the nurse's station, where I dialed my home number. Tom would just be waking up. I hoped he wasn't in the shower. The phone rang three times, then I heard his voice. "Dr. Harman," he answered good-naturedly.

Back in the birthing room, I glanced at the monitor. No decelerations, fetal heart rate 130 with accelerations up to 150; it couldn't be better. The contractions, however, were lame. They came every three minutes, but by palpation were only moderate. Amber's uterus was pooped, and it wouldn't help to increase the IV drip.

"Watch your eyes, Amber and Darrell," I said. "I'm going to turn up the lights. It's time to have a baby. Dr. Harman will be here in about 20 minutes to help with the vacuum and I want to be ready."

Amber looked at me with big eyes when I mentioned the vacuum, but she didn't resist. I checked her one more time. The little head was still sitting exactly where it had been for the last hour.

Twenty minutes later, Tom Harman strolled into the room in blue scrubs. I'd braided Amber's long auburn hair, washed her face, fluffed up her pillow, and given her a clean top sheet. Our nurse, Nancy, had turned on the infant warmer and readied the delivery table.

Tom approached the bed gently, nodded to Darrell, glanced at the fetal monitor, and rested his hand on Amber's foot. He looked into her eyes and smiled. "Time to have a baby? Want some help?"

That's what I liked about working with my husband. He never acted like Superman coming in to save the day, never made a woman feel like a failure. He was just there to assist however we needed him.

I explained the vacuum extractor to the young couple: "It's a small plastic suction cup that fits on the baby's head. When Tom pulls, you have to push, Amber. It's a two-person job. When you run out of air, go back down again quick."

The doctor and I were now gloved and gowned. The room was crackling with the electricity. "Come on, Amber. Push!" we all entreated. Tom applied steady downward traction to bring the fetal head under the pubic bone; the vacuum popped off.

This isn't going to be easy. By protocol we have three tries. Any more can be dangerous.

Another long, steady pull and the suction cup popped off again. The top of the baby's head was almost crowning, but despite everyone's effort, the hairy orb slipped back into the vagina.

We had one more try. *If this doesn't work, we'll have to do a C-section.* I swallowed hard. "Let's go, Amber. Push like your life depended on it." The next thing I knew, the head was crowning for real. Tom removed the vacuum and I poured oil over his gloved fingers as he eased the vaginal tissues back.

"You are on your own now, Amber. Go ahead and have your baby." One more big push, and the baby slid out.

I wasn't alarmed by the infant's weak cry. What startled me was the shape of her head. It was not only molded, but the soft, squishy caput was over one of the parietal bones. Amber reached out when the nurse handed her the baby, wrapped snuggly in double receiving blankets, with a white knit cap over her head. "Oh Emily," she cried. "My Emily."

Darrell had tears in his eyes, and I did too. Tom put his arm around me; another nice birth, not easy, or uncomplicated, but nice. The light in the room was golden.

After charting and signing the birth certificate, I canceled my patients in the office, went home for a few hours of sleep, then returned for afternoon clinic. It wasn't until six P.M. that I got back to Community Hospital to make rounds.

I stopped first at the nurses' station to review my patient's vital signs. I was surprised to find the chart already broken down with a discharge instruction sheet lying on top. "What's up?" I asked Mrs. Bartola, nodding at Amber's chart and frowning at the ward secretary, who was drowning in a sea of paperwork.

She brushed two strands of her long, gray hair back. "Your patient wants to be discharged," Mrs. Bartola snapped. "She's been waiting for you to make rounds."

I sighed and sat down. "I was up all night, then had patients in the office. Anyway, it's too early for her to go home. The pediatricians will want to keep the newborn for at least 24 hours. She's not leaving without her baby."

"That's why she wants out of here. The infant was transferred, by ambulance, to the NICU at the University Hospital six hours ago. She wants to get over there."

"What!" I almost jump out of my chair. "Why didn't they call me?"

"It's been a zoo around here. Four deliveries this morning. It's slowing down now. Someone tried. I think they left a message on your home phone. "

"Well, what *happened*?" The secretary shrugged as if this didn't concern her. She was just there for the paycheck.

"Ask Nancy; she's the charge nurse."

I found the RN in the nursery cleaning an empty infant warmer. "So, what happened to Amber's baby?" I started out without preamble.

Nancy turned, but didn't stop wiping.

"*You know*, little Emily, in 605. Amber and Darrell's baby, born this morning at 7:30, remember? The kid with the funny cone head. She was fine when I left."

"Oh," Nancy responded. "That one. We've had so many. She was shipped to Children's, across town, for seizure precautions. Cara was in the nursery and thought the baby was trembling and then it rolled its eyes. She's a new grad, a little nervous.

"When she called Dr. Jenkins, the peds on call, he said, 'Ship her.' Had an office full of sick kids with the flu. It's probably just as well. We're full to capacity and don't have a spare nurse to sit in the nursery. All the other babies are in the birthing rooms with their moms."

I was not sympathetic. Maybe I should have been, but I wondered about Cara's judgment. It wasn't a big deal to the staff if baby Emily was separated from her parents, but to Amber and Darrell it was. On the other hand, if something was seriously wrong, the infant was better off in the NICU with the close observation of experienced nurses and neonatologists.

I shuffled, with heavy feet, down the long carpeted hall to room 605, where Amber was sitting dressed in street clothes, talking on her cell phone. "Got to go,

Mom," she signed off. Darrell came out of the bathroom. Their suitcases were packed at the door.

I began by apologizing. "I would have come right to the hospital or discharged you over the phone if I'd known what happened, but I didn't get the message." Then I gave the young woman her postpartum instructions and a hug. "I'm sure the baby will be okay," I told her. "But don't forget to take care of yourself. If you get sick or run down, you won't be able to take care of Emily when she comes home."

At eight the next morning, as I stood at Emily's clear plastic–enclosed bed in the NICU, I was puzzled. *This doesn't look like the same infant I delivered 24 hours ago.* There was an oxygen tube in her nose and an IV in her head. Monitor leads were taped all over her chest. Except for her color, which was pale pink, she looked like death warmed over. The white knit cap still covered her caput.

I caught Mattie, the NICU nurse's, eye. We knew each other from when I used to work as a faculty nurse-midwife at University Hospital. "What's up with Emily?"

Mattie put her hand on the plastic infant bed, as tenderly as if touching the child. "Just seizure precautions. She's on a phenobarbital drip." The RN leaned close. "Anything happen at the birth?" I winced.

"No. Not really. It was a long second stage and a vacuum delivery, but not unusual. The fetal heart tracing was fine. Apgar scores, 7–9. Are Emily's parents around?"

"They were here all night and finally went home to sleep. Real nice people."

My plan was to come back at six after clinic, but I had a delivery instead. I wasn't home until midnight and didn't make it back to the NICU until eight the following morning. This time I found Amber sitting in a rocking chair, stroking her baby's face through the portholes. Emily still looked the same: pale pink, inert, barely alive. I glanced up at the monitors over her bed, then sat down beside the young mother. "So what do the pediatricians say? Does Emily ever fuss or cry? Can you breastfeed her?" I skipped the pleasantries.

"No, she doesn't do anything. They don't know what's wrong. She was okay when I last saw her at the Birthing Center, but after she went to the nursery and had the seizure there was no response. She's getting a brain scan this afternoon."

I stuck out my jaw as if somehow I could *will* this baby to be okay, then stepped closer to look. Emily was a tiny sleeping beauty. The pointy-head was now round, with soft black curls. She was the prettiest infant in the NICU and the only one that was full term. *Why is she just lying there? Why isn't she squirming or rooting for food?*

"Do they let you hold her?"

"Not yet. Maybe tonight, after the brain scan. They don't want to stimulate her too much." Seizures are a sign of brain injury or swelling. I wasn't sure if the mother knew this, but now was not the time to explain. She was worried enough already.

I gave Amber a hug and asked her to call me on my cell if there was a change, for better or worse, and then

I went looking for a resident to get a report. Dr. Cooma's summary was not what I wanted to hear.

"We think the baby's a gork," he told me after I introduced myself. This young man had no idea what that word mean to a parent, or to a midwife or physician who delivered the baby, but I didn't reprimand him.

"What's the next step?"

"Brain scan this evening. Then transfer her to Step Down. She's breathing fine. Oxygen saturation is normal. She just won't eat or do anything else. Probably send the kid home on phenobarb and a monitor. There's not much else we can do."

"There's no chance the phenobarbital is sedating her too much?"

The resident's pager was going off and he looked at the number and shrugged. "Naw, half these kids are on phenobarb. Routine."

At home, I told my husband the situation over a dinner of pork chops and salad, then retreated to my study. *I don't understand it. The baby was fine when I left the Birthing Center a few hours after birth.* I pored through my old maternal child nursing books. Nothing was helpful. I checked out the baby's medication in an old copy of the *Physician's Desk Reference*, skimming through "Dosage" and "Drug Interactions" to get to "Side Effects." "Drowsiness" was the first one mentioned.

No, I concluded. The NICU nurses and doctors knew what they were doing. Thousands of babies got this medicine without ill effect.

By the weekend, Emily had been moved to Step Down. Her IV had been removed and she was getting formula and breast milk by nasogastric tube. I visited every day, sometimes in the morning, sometimes at night. Emily and Darrell continued their vigil at the unresponsive baby's bedside. Her flaccid, beautiful slumbering body was a mystery. I asked the mother, "Does she *ever* respond to you? Hold your finger or anything? Has she had any more seizures?"

"She opens her eyes sometimes when I touch her. I think that she focuses. I think that she sees me, but then she closes them again. She hasn't had any seizures since they transferred her from Community Hospital."

It wasn't my intention to cause my patient to doubt her caregivers' wisdom, but I couldn't help myself. "Amber, I've been thinking about the phenobarbital. You know, the medicine the baby's getting for seizure precautions? That drug causes drowsiness, makes you very sleepy. Do you think that could be the problem? I've asked the doctors and nurses, but you're the baby's mother. Could you ask again? See if they'll take the dose down. They might listen to you. If the baby actually has a seizure, they could always go up again." Emily swallowed. I could see the idea interested her, but she was afraid. When you're a parent with a very sick baby, it's hard to challenge the experts.

As I left, my friend Robin, a nurse practitioner, caught me by the lab coat sleeve and pulled me into her tiny office. "Patsy," she said, "Emily's brain scan was normal, but the ECG isn't. I just thought I should tell you.

We're going to have a patient conference with the family tonight: the neonatologist, the chief resident, the nurse, and I. We have to let Amber and Darrell know that Emily has no capacity for normal life. Her basic reflexes are gone. She'll probably be discharged home, soon, with an apnea monitor."

"It couldn't be the phenobarb, could it?" I tried one more time. Robin shook her head no, as if to say, "Give it up, Patsy."

I was sick with remorse. Maybe we should have done a C-section. I was crushed for the family.

In the morning, I returned to the NICU before office hours with a heavy heart, unsure what I'd find. Amber and Darrell would have been informed of the infant's grave prognosis. I expected to see the young parents crying at the baby's bedside.

Instead, I found Amber sitting in a rocking chair, holding Emily, who was sucking eagerly at a bottle with milk dribbling down her chin. Her eyes were wide open and when Amber took the bottle away, the baby rooted eagerly.

"*What happened?*" I asked, astounded. Amber looked around and then said in a low voice, "I did what you said. I insisted they take the baby off the phenobarb for one night. In the morning a new neonatologist came on duty, Dr. Hatch."

"I know Dr. Hatch, she's a no-nonsense woman. All the nurses and residents are afraid of her."

"*No*, she's really nice. She walked up to Emily's bed and said, 'Why isn't this baby eating?' The RN tried to explain that Emily *couldn't* eat; she couldn't even swallow. But Dr. Hatch said, '*Nonsense*. You aren't trying hard enough!'

"I don't know if it was stopping the phenobarb or just everyone putting in more effort, but the nurse took the baby and gave her the bottle. At first we had to stroke Emily's cheek and her throat to get her to swallow and suck, but now she's eating just fine."

Amber stared down at her baby with pride, the same way she looked at the infant right after birth. I didn't know whether to laugh or to cry, so I did both. The color of the room turned golden again.

Emily, like Lazarus, had risen from the grave.

Voyagers

~

Julianna Paradisi, RN

Survival is grim for a newborn unable to breathe the air of the planet he is born on.

Before his birth, he was an aquanaut, floating in amniotic fluid inside his mother's womb. Inside that dark, familiar space, he thrived. However, once he left it, things immediately went amiss.

The system malfunction occurred during the early weeks of his mother's pregnancy. The apparatus of his heart did not work. In turn, his lungs became diseased. At birth, no longer tethered by his umbilical cord to the life support of a placenta, he began dying as soon as he reached the bright lights of the delivery room. He was unable to breathe Earth's atmosphere. A breathing tube placed in his throat saved him. It connected to a ventilator, his new life support system. Then he was loaded into a helicopter, and arrived at our hospital from out of the sky, akin to The Little Prince in Saint-Exupéry's book. Charming and precious (the proof of his existence), he may as well have been from outer space, for his inability to survive on our planet.

I was his nurse in the Pediatric Intensive Care Unit, following his cardiac surgery. Persistently, his lungs refused to adapt. A canister the size of a full-grown person bled nitric oxide into the ventilator tubes, blending it with oxygen in an effort to coax the lungs into functioning. He had other problems too. The surgical repair of his heart went well, but the surgeon could not close the incision in the newborn's chest. Inflammation and swelling are the body's normal response to surgery, and fluids pumped through the bypass machine into his veins to keep him stable contributed to the problem. Between the two, there was too much swelling for the surgeon to close the chest. Instead, a transparent dressing stretched over the surgical site, covering it in much the same way as plastic wrap covers a bowl of fruit salad. His walnut-sized heart was visible as it beat in the chest underneath the dressing. I was unnerved the first time I saw a baby return from the OR like this. I can only imagine what it did to his parents. Before they saw him in the PICU, the surgeon explained that the open chest was temporary, until the edema subsided. This could take a day or a week or two, but then he would close the chest. A case manager talked to them too, explaining what they would see, and answered their questions. Inside the PICU room, I placed a thin receiving blanket over his chest. Printed with yellow bunnies (I know that blue brings out the dusky color of the baby's skin, and is not complimentary), it is often the only item in the hospital room suggesting the idea of a nursery. I do not remove it in the parents' presence unless they ask me to. Many parents choose to look under the blanket. They take inventory of what they see, and I study the expressions on their faces while the fragments of a shattered dream rain upon them. The first question is always, "Is he in pain?" I reassured them their newborn was receiving continuous IV infusions of strong narcotics and sedatives to prevent pain. I told them I would look for signs of breakthrough pain, and their doctor had ordered more pain medications if it occured. I explained the baby was motionless because he also received a paralytic medication so he would not move and aggravate the healing process. Only the ever-present monitor screen with its tracings of heartbeat and respirations was proof that their baby was still alive. They did not have any more questions. They did not stay long. Later, for the sake of their baby, they would learn to see past the open chest and the tubes. They would learn to look for signs of improvement, but not on the first visit.

My small patient lay on his back, naked except for a disposable diaper. He lay on a mattress supported by a platform with four Plexiglas sides. Above it was a warming light that read a heart-shaped, gold-foil sensor adhered to his torso. The sensor monitored the newborn's body temperature and the light adjusted the amount of radiant heat by its settings. It warmed the baby without blankets so I could see him at all times. On one of his big toes was the red light of a pulse ox, and I thought of ET's glowing finger. "Home," I said to no one in particular. Hinges on the Plexiglas sides allowed me to adjust tubes, monitor leads, and change the linen without moving the baby. Next to the warmer was a ventilator, connected to the baby's breathing tube. Beside it stood the looming canister of nitric oxide. Three IV poles held seven IV infusion pumps and several mini infusion pumps. A chest tube bubbled water in a plastic box hanging from the warmer. His parents joked it was their son's water feature, an effort toward something familiar. Because of the shock to his body from the crash delivery and surgery, his kidneys were sluggish. Peritoneal dialysis removed toxins from his body, because he did not make enough pee. A Foley catheter threaded into his penis and draining urine into a bag confirmed that finding. From another IV pole hung the three-liter bag of dialysate. Everything connected by tubes to the baby. The cardiac monitor glowed green on the wall above. He no longer wore a receiving blanket over his open chest; his parents realized that this was not his most serious problem. They did not want the blanket obstructing my view of their son or his life-sustaining, artificial, environment. Under the bright lights, surrounded by all of this technology, lay a newborn weighing six and a half pounds and only 19 inches tall, the price of surviving in another world.

I spent my shift in his room, checking settings, replacing used fluid bags, and giving medications. I remembered to talk to him softly and to touch him gently. My patient was, after all, a baby.

Through the windows of his room, I noticed two women in suits enter the PICU. They stopped in the hall at the door of the room and looked inside. I recognized one of the women as the director of the children's hospital. I did not know the other one, but later learned she was one of its senior administrators. From the doorway, they said a brief hello to me, and turned away to discuss, presumably, our PICU. Then they walked on. Moments later, the woman I did not know came back to the doorway, but did not enter. She took a long, sweeping look. Her eyes took in the equipment, pumps, and monitors, and then came to rest on the warmer. "My God," she asked, incredulously, "is that a baby in there?"

I almost laughed at her. I wanted to say, "Yes, this is a baby. Come in and see. Look at his open chest. Come in and see what I do. I juggle complex tasks so everything works, and nothing goes wrong. Come in, and see what his parents see daily. Think about the pain they feel. This is what we do in this unit, in this hospital. Think about this when you make your reports and budgets."

I did not say any of this. I just nodded. She shook her head sadly and walked away, in her suit and pumps. I stood there in my scrubs and clogs, comprehending that she and I are creatures from segregated galaxies of the same universe. She was an alien in this room, just as I would be in her boardroom, if I had to present a budget or report to the CEO. This baby was the sky bridge that joined us. He was the reason we maintained this spaceship called a hospital. If she failed her job, the hospital would malfunction, and I could not do mine. Without me, her job did not matter. We do not speak the same language and we do not look alike, this administrator and I. Sometimes our relationship is adversarial. This encounter reminded me of our need to find ways to work together, so patients like this voyager get the care they need, and deserve. There are two kinds of jobs in a hospital: one makes decisions how to run it, and the other provides the care. Rarely do the two meet in a patient's room.

The Inseparable Unit

~

Barbara Latterner, BSN, RN, IBCLC

THE CUTTING OF the umbilical cord tends to herald the arrival of a new and unique life. Though this tiny being began its existence many months before, growing nestled and protected within the womb, the just-born infant is seen as an individual apart from his or her mother. There is, however, a significant error in this thinking, for baby and mother are one, so to speak, and severing this unit denies an empirical truth. Birth should not be a celebration of separation, but rather a reuniting of mother and baby, who joins her for an external connection.

It is upon this premise that I base my practice as a lactation consultant. The importance of mother/baby togetherness is a familiar mantra of mine from prenatal breastfeeding classes to individual private-practice home visits, to weekly mom-and-baby groups. At the core of my work with infants is respect for each baby as an individual, as well as the "partner" of his/her mother in an important and inseparable dyad. Breastfeeding is a mutual function of both baby and mother, obviously affecting one another. The infant who has difficulty correctly sucking may damage his mother's nipples, for example, and the mother who unknowingly positions her baby too far from her breast may also cause herself nipple pain and lessen the amount of food her baby receives. One cannot treat an infant with breastfeeding difficulties without including the mother, nor should other situations necessitating nursing care of the infant neglect to include the mother.

In the past almost 19 years of working with breastfeeding infants and their mothers, first as a La Leche League leader and then as a certified, professional lactation consultant, I have experienced many situations of intense involvement with breastfeeding dyads. None compare, however, to the most intimate and personal one of my own daughter and grandson. Christopher Thomas was born at 34½ weeks' gestation via cesarean section and his early days of life were unfortunately spent, for the most part, separated from his mother. Despite the fact that he arrived breathing well on his own, receiving Apgars of 8 and 9, he was soon taken to the neonatal intensive care unit, where intravenous fluids were started.

Present throughout my daughter Jennifer's C-section, I basically stood there in shock, witnessing a surgery on my eldest I wish I hadn't. Her midwife, who was present as well, at one point noticed my near shocklike state, asking,

"Are you all right, Barbara? You're looking rather pale." No wonder, for events happened all too fast and this unplanned surgery due to lack of labor progression was taking its toll.

Her arms strapped to boards in extension, and medicated to vague awareness, Jennifer's initial contact with her infant son was limited to cheek-to-cheek contact thoughtfully provided by her midwife, who held Christopher close to his mother, telling her what a beautiful baby she had. Several minutes of debate between the midwife and the neonatologist regarding my grandson's fate ensued. The midwife felt Christopher was healthily responsive and belonged with his mother, while the neonatologist preferred to admit him to the NICU due to the numbers (gestational age). Unfortunately, the neonatologist's opinion prevailed regardless of signs to the contrary—weight of five pounds, eight ounces, all vital signs within normal limits, and an alert little one in no apparent distress. Lacking professional expertise with newly born premature infants, and feeling overwhelmed due to my personal involvement, I stood helplessly by as my precious grandson was taken away.

Could Christopher have been put on his mother's chest, for even a short while, to stabilize his major life functions and normalize his first extra-uterine experiences? Do I now regret not requesting this as my daughter and grandson's advocate? Most definitely! Was infant observation warranted? Yes. Could this have been done without separation? Most likely. Harsh as this may sound, I'm afraid that a newly opened Level III nursery, with Christopher about to become their first patient, may have influenced this and subsequent decisions about his care.

How much of my grandson's treatment was appropriate or even necessary is sadly debatable, and my doubts and criticism may be construed as a grandmother's usual protectiveness. However, my daughter and I, who tentatively questioned then, and now more confidently question in hindsight, were not the only ones who felt a different course of action could have been taken. Professional friends and colleagues, including physicians and lactation consultants (some who actually examined Christopher or worked with him), expressed their doubts about the reasons for his lengthy hospitalization.

My sweet grandson, during his 11-day stay in the NICU, underwent unnecessary invasive testing (IVs, heel sticks, a spinal tap), but worst of all, Jennifer and Christopher suffered the absolute agony of separation from one another. I saw it myself in Christopher's behavior as he struggled to gain comfort in cotton blankets and bolsters, alone in his plastic box, and I saw it in my daughter's tearful eyes as she touched her son's long fingers, desperate to hold him for more than some designated times. I remember nighttime calls from Jennifer, after I went home from my daily, daylong hospital visits, tearfully reporting the evening's events, wishing she were home with her baby. Even today, four years later, Jennifer expresses her doubts and guilt about what transpired. After validating her feelings, I remind her of her admirable bravery, persistence, and strong motherly instincts that kept her by her baby's side. Once her allotted days for C-section recovery were over, I recall her stating adamantly, "I'm staying in the hospital with Christopher, even if I have to sleep in a chair in the NICU. I will not go home and leave my baby alone." Fortunately, due to low census and an understanding hospital lactation consultant and nursing staff, she was given a private room.

As soon as she was "allowed" (not soon enough in my opinion), she began kangaroo care, skin-to-skin contact with her son. Always stable, often blissfully sleeping, it was apparent that Christopher was where he'd belonged all along, safe and nurtured, on his mother's chest. Photos were taken of this precious time, and the strained look on my daughter's face as she tried to contain her tears haunts me still. Her loss of early mothering normalcy was being grieved, and though mostly resolved emotionally, she continues to mourn this loss, and like other mothers like her, always will.

More difficult to quantify is Christopher's early emotional trauma due to the initial separation from his mother, in addition to the painful procedures he underwent. Hopefully assuaged by barely interrupted physical contact with his mother once he was home, and her frequent apologies to him, whispered amid her kisses and tears, my dear grandchild has weathered well his stormy beginning.

Breastfeeding, while providing more physical contact and loving warmth, was unfortunately fraught with difficulties due to Christopher's poor oral tone. Since he was unable to suck correctly, exclusive breastfeeding was not possible, but breastmilk was given by various alternative feeding methods. Although Jennifer religiously expressed her milk by routine pumping, her condition of insulin resistance, part of the polycystic ovarian syndrome she was diagnosed with later, interfered with her ability to provide for all of Christopher's nutritional needs. Donor milk was obtained to complement his required intake. Christopher, despite outside expert lactation consultant help, as well as speech and occupational therapies, was able to breastfeed only partially for several months, while donor milk supplemented Jennifer's almost two years of pumping for her son.

Obviously, there is more to this story than is detailed here, as I am focusing on the one aspect of unnecessary infant/mother separation. So why didn't I, the experienced lactation consultant and nurse, act on my suspicions of my grandson's unnecessary hospitalization? I think I was fearful of acting rashly, unsure of my own judgment in this situation, but also was being respectful of the fact that this was my daughter's child and her decision to make. Christopher, diagnosed with global motor planning deficit and apraxia of speech, continues to have hurdles to overcome. I will always regretfully wonder whether the early separation from his mother had to be one of those hurdles.

Due to my dear daughter's strong belief in the importance of attachment parenting and hard work, Christopher is an intelligent, connected, and happy child whose sense of humor and resiliency brings me much joy. My work with breastfeeding dyads continues to reflect what I learned from this experience: Babies belong with their mothers. As tempting as it may be sometimes to personally guide that baby to breast, I sit on my hands to let his mother do it herself, guiding instead with words of instruction and encouragement. I am also quick to point out to each mom how much her baby likes and needs her: "See how she smiles at you and turns to your voice?" "See how content your little one is snuggled in your arms or sleeping on your chest?" Opportunities abound for nurturing mother/baby togetherness. I also do not forget the wise and intelligent words of Dr. James McKenna, who states, "The mother is the environment for her baby."

Acknowledgment of Permissions

"In god's palm" is reprinted with the kind permission of Nancy Leigh Harless. The story originally appeared in *Womankind: Connection and Wisdom Around the World*, released by Tate Enterprises October 2007.

Reader's Guide

1. Amy and her baby, Adam, taught Carole Kenner that if she didn't take care of the family, she didn't take care of the baby. Looking back, Carole says, "In my quest to master the clinical complexities of an intensive care setting, I was still on a learning curve when integrating the holistic and psychological/social aspects of nursing care." Do you remember when you first became aware of the importance of integrating these two aspects of patient care? If so, how did that moment change the way you practiced nursing?

2. In "A Gut Feeling," Dianna Hannah knew something was wrong with baby Sam: though he ultimately didn't survive, her insistence that the other nurses more thoroughly examine Sam enabled them to catch his respiratory distress immediately. Her story illustrates the importance of respecting your gut feelings, and asking questions of more experienced nurses and doctors without fear of annoying them. Have you ever had a gut feeling about a patient? What did you do about it?

3. Cara Bicking describes how other nurses were uncomfortable with the parents' decision to take their baby home to die rather than allow him to continue curative care in "When a Baby's Short Life Is at Home." How do you handle yourself when your patient makes a decision you disagree with? Are you honest, do you lie, or do you avoid the issue? Compare and contrast the nurses' behavior and the parents' responses in Cara's essay to those in "Better Late Than Never" by Dawn M. Kersula.

4. The majority of stories in this collection, and perhaps in life, revolve around the basic assumption that a baby belongs with its parents, particularly with its mother. In some stories, giving a baby time with its parents was a crucial part of the healing process for all, even when the infant did not survive. But in "David's Miracle," the authorities ultimately decide that the baby of a severe alcoholic will be better off with an adopted family than with its own mother. Can you think of other instances in which it is not in the baby's best interest to be with his or her family? What other reasons might there be for such a decision?

5. In "Stolen Time" Margie Marier-Porchia describes her disappointment that she had denied a prematurely born baby precious moments with his parents while she and other nurses were taking notes and making plans for his care. Do you think they were wrong to

monitor him and make such plans given his condition? How do you know when it is time to fight and when it is more important to give a family time to be together?

6. Religion plays a role in many of these stories. In some, like "In God's Palm," it is a source of strength and a coping mechanism in the face of ignorance and poverty. In others, like "Changing Assignments," it provides comfort and acceptance that we can't control everything. Discuss how religion has influenced or otherwise played a role in your own cases. How has it helped patients or nurses cope? Has religion ever played a negative part in a patient's situation?

7. As have many medical professionals before her, Karen Klein felt confident that her experience as a nurse would help her to be a better mother to her newborn infant. Explain what she means when she says that she was "so used to dealing with very sick people that I was not as easily alarmed as a parent who wasn't a nurse might be." Why does she conclude that being a nurse won't necessarily make you an exemplary caregiver to your own child or loved one? Do you agree or disagree? How else might being a nurse become a detriment rather than a benefit?

8. The nurses in this collection emphasize that caring for neonatal infants is a vocation filled with as

much heartache as there is joy. What kind of balance between the two have you experienced in your own work? Does the joy outweigh the heartache for you? What is "burnout" and how do you recognize it? How can you protect yourself from "burnout"?

9. In the course of a nursing career, there will be births, deaths, and recoveries that change your life forever. Share with your book club one story of a patient you will never forget. Have you stayed in touch with this, or any other, patient? What prompts you to build a relationship with some discharged patients and not others? Do you feel it is professional for a nurse to become personally involved with her patients both in and beyond the hospital?

10. Ideally, doctors and nurses work closely together to provide the best possible care for their patients. But the nurses in these stories often express feelings of frustration with the doctors involved in their cases. Do you agree that it is a nurse's job to challenge and push the doctors on their patients' behalf? How does this role conflict with the nurse's job as a hospital team member? Is it ever okay to share your opinion with patients when it goes against the doctor's opinion, as Patricia Harman does in "Emily"? How do you decide when to challenge the experts and when to support the hospital's decisions?

11. J. Paradisi likens the hospital to a spaceship populated with segregated life-forms. The administrators who run the place are seldom connected to the people who provide care to the patients. Have you experienced a situation in which you felt a "suit" was too alien to the situation to make a good decision? Discuss the ways in which communication between hospital staff and administration has worked or not worked in your hospital and identify some possible solutions.

12. In "The Inseparable Unit," Barbara Latterner quotes Dr. James McKenna as saying that "the mother is the environment for her baby." But when infants are separated from their mothers for intensive care, as they often are in this book, their environment becomes the hospital and the "plastic box" of the NICU. How do you think this environment affects the babies? Have you ever had the opportunity to observe a former NICU baby later in life and identified behaviors that you think were influenced by this very early separation?

About the Editor

For more than 35 years, **Kathleen Huggins, RN, MS,** has dedicated her medical career to helping mothers care more effectively for their newborn babies. Kathleen is a registered nurse and has a master's degree in Perinatal Nursing from University of California, San Francisco. She moved to San Luis Obispo in 1980 with her young daughter to work at San Luis Obispo General Hospital. Quickly she became a community resource for breast-feeding mothers. In 1983, she founded the Breastfeeding Warmline, a telephone counseling service, and soon after, one of the first breastfeeding clinics in the country.

Kathleen authored *The Nursing Mother's Companion* in 1986, which quickly became a bestseller. It is now in its fifth edition and has sold more than 1,000,000 copies. She gave birth to her second child and wrote a second book, *The Nursing Mother's Guide to Weaning*.

Kathleen directed the San Luis Obispo Breastfeeding Clinic for more than 20 years until her diagnosis of breast cancer and her retirement in 2004. In 2002, Kathleen opened Simply MaMa, a maternity and nursing boutique in downtown San Luis. She leads seminars on a variety of topics related to perinatal care and breastfeeding. She lives with her husband and son in San Luis Obispo.

About the Contributors

LANETTE L. ANDERSON, MSN, JD, RN, is the executive director of the West Virginia State Board of Examiners for Licensed Practical Nurses. She has been employed with the Board since 1992, and has been the ED since 2001. She has been licensed as a registered nurse since 1980, and completed a master's in Nursing Administration in 2006. Her clinical practice includes working as a staff nurse in a Level III Neonatal ICU for several years. Anderson graduated from law school at West Virginia University in 1992 and has been licensed as an attorney in the state of West Virginia since that time. She has served on a variety of committees with the National Council of State Boards of Nursing, and currently is serving on committees for the Council on Licensure, Enforcement, and Regulation. Anderson is also an adjunct faculty member in the LPN to BSN program at Mountain State University, the BSN program at Kaplan University, and the MSN program at Olivet Nazarene University, primarily teaching leadership, legal issues, and ethics. She also is a regular contributing author to www.nursetogether.com.

CARA BICKING, RNC, BSN, is a staff nurse in the Neonatal Intensive Care Unit of the Penn State Hershey Children's Hospital in Hershey, Pennsylvania. She is a graduate of Juniata College in Huntingdon, Pennsylvania, as well as of Thomas Jefferson University in Philadelphia, Pennsylvania. She anticipates the completion of her master's degree in Nursing Education from Walden University in March of 2009.

CAROL BLAIR-MURDOCH, RN, BSCN, has enjoyed nursing children since 1986, commencing her career in Toronto at the Hospital for Sick Children in their Cardiology unit. Throughout her nursing years she took several contracts in Saudi Arabia in both Pediatric and Neonatal Intensive Care units. She enjoyed several months of travel on either end of those contracts. Currently she lives with her husband and two children in Mississauga, Canada. She enjoys the balance and challenge of working as a part-time clinical educator in a Special Care Nursery at the community hospital near her home and continuing as a part-time nurse at the bedside in the Cardiac Critical Care Unit at the Hospital for Sick Children.

SUZANNA M. FELICIANO, BSN, RN, CCRN, has been employed at University Health Systems, San Antonio, Texas, since 1978. Currently, she is a Staff Nurse III in NICU. Her nursing experience includes work in General Pediatrics, PICU (Cardiac/Renal/Trauma Unit), and the Post Anesthesia Care Unit. She has published two articles in the *Journal of Perioperative Nursing*: "Infant Heart Transplantation" in January 1992, and "Ross-Kono Procedure" in April 1995. In 2008, she served as the conference chair for the Texas Association of PeriAnesthesia Nurses State Conference.

MONICA FROMMER, RN is a registered nurse specializing in newborn and maternal postpartum healthcare as well as a private in-hospital nurse. She offers a variety of services ranging from prenatal consulting, postpartum hospital care, and postpartum home care via her website, www.mommyandbabynurse.com.

DIANNA M. HANNAH, RN, is a registered nurse on a busy postpartum floor and well-baby nursery at Mary Washington Hospital in Fredericksburg, Virginia. She feels blessed to have a job she loves and especially enjoys teaching and spending time with new parents. Dianna grew up in Baltimore, Maryland, where she earned her nursing degree at Catonsville Community College in 1998. She now resides in Spotsylvania, Virginia, where she's lived for nine years with her husband and two sons.

NANCY LEIGH HARLESS, ARNP, is an award-winning poet, writer, and women's healthcare nurse practitioner. Her works have been included in many anthologies including *Travelers' Tales, Cup of Comfort, The Healing Project,* and *Chicken Soup for the Soul.* Recently retired, Harless travels often—usually off the well-paved road. Throughout her travels she has seen women struggle, sometimes against daunting odds. She has seen them nearly break under the weight of their own lives. She also has felt an abundance of spirit, of wisdom, and of connection with these same women—ordinary women who live with extraordinary grace. Their stories make up her recently released book, *Womankind: Connection & Wisdom Around the World* (www.womankindconnection.com).

PATRICIA HARMAN, RN, CNM, MSN, is the author of *The Blue Cotton Gown: A Midwife's Memoir* (Beacon Press, 2008). She is a graduate of the University of Minnesota, St. Joseph's College in Maine, and Hocking College in Ohio and has been a nurse for 25 years. She is on the clinical faculty of West Virginia University School of Nursing and works in private practice with her husband, an ob-gyn in Morgantown, West Virginia.

NICOLE M. JARRELL, MSN, RNC, has 18 years of neonatal and pediatric cardiac intensive care nursing. Currently, her role is as a system clinical nurse specialist for an integrated five-hospital system. She has a BSN from Medical University of South Carolina and an MSN from University of Phoenix. A special thanks to her wonderful husband for his support and encouragement. And to all the babies and families who hold a piece of her heart.

BONNIE JARVIS-LOWE, RN, is a 60-year-old retired registered nurse who worked in various hospitals across Canada. She retired at age 51 to return to her home province of Newfoundland and Labrador with her retired policeman husband. She has been practicing and enjoying her homeland, photography, and writing since retirement. She has two adult children and one grandchild in western Canada, and misses them terribly.

CAROLE KENNER, DNS, RNC-NIC, FAAN, is a dean and professor at the University of Oklahoma. Dr. Kenner received her BSN from the University of Cincinnati and her master's and doctorate from Indiana University. She has over 25 years' experience in education at all levels of nursing—BSN through PhD. Dr. Kenner has presented on local, state, national, and international levels regarding neonatal/perinatal/genetic/core care. She is president of the Council of International Neonatal Nurses, Inc. and serves on the Nursing Advisory Board, National March of Dimes.

DAWN M. KERSULA, MA, RN, FACCE, IBCLC, is a perinatal educator and lactation consultant at Brattleboro Memorial Hospital in Brattleboro, Vermont. She has been helping moms and babies breastfeed happily for over 25 years, and currently speaks to audiences of nurses around the country about the nuts and bolts of breastfeeding support. Her master's degree study looked at the experience of PTSD for mothers who experienced trauma during the birth of a baby.

KAREN KLEIN, RN, obtained her BSN from Adelphi University, graduating magna cum laude. Her varied nursing experience includes ER/Trauma, Pediatrics,

Interventional Radiology, Telemetry, ICU, Home Infusion, and Occupational Health. She is a certified emergency nurse and an American Heart Association CPR/first aid instructor, and has been published by *Nursing Spectrum Magazine.*

VERA KNOX, RNC, was born and raised near the Neandertal in Germany. She came to the United States in 1982 and has been a labor and delivery nurse at Palomar Medical Center, Escondido, California, for the last 23 years. Of all the strange, sad, and wonderful experiences she has had during that time, she considers "The Cath Lab Baby" the most memorable.

BARBARA LATTERNER, BSN, RN, IBCLC, graduated from Creighton University in 1970. Initial practice as an RN included NICU, pediatrics, and psychiatric nursing in staff, supervisory, and educational roles. Interest in breastfeeding began with the nursing of her three daughters and the joining of La Leche League, serving as a leader from 1989 to 1996. She has been board certified as a lactation consultant since 1996 when she began her private practice, in which she continues to passionately and respectfully provide for mothers and babies.

KELLY MAIDMENT, RN, resides in Ottawa, Canada, and has been an RN for 14 years, having worked in many areas including the emergency department. After a high-risk pregnancy, her son spent time in the NICU. When she returned from maternity leave, she began working in the same NICU where her son had been a patient, and still works at the Ottawa Hospital-General campus, in a 26-bed Level III NICU.

MARGIE MARIER-PORCHIA, RN, BS, graduated in 1991, receiving national certification as a NIDCAP observer in 2005. She presently works as a bedside nurse, transport nurse, and NIDCAP observer at a Level III NICU at St. Luke's Regional Medical Center in Boise, Idaho. She has received the March of Dimes Regional Pediatric Nurse of the Year Award (2007) and recently presented her shared research on the effect of relationship-based care on RN job satisfaction at the WINN conference (2008). Her husband, two children, and family are the inspiration in her life.

JULIANNA PARADISI, RN, finds inspiration when science, humanity, and art converge. She works to create compelling images as both a writer and a painter. A nurse for 22 years, she has worked in Pediatric Intensive Care in Level III trauma centers in California and Oregon. A cancer survivor, she credits her pediatric patients with teaching her how to behave herself when it hurts. Now working in adult oncology, she lives with her husband in Portland, Oregon.

ROBIN A. ROOTS, RN, IBCLC, has always been interested in writing, and during her college years had a story published in her college paper. She was considering pursuing an English major. However, her desire to be more involved with helping people led her to pursue a career in nursing. She has never regretted that decision. At the age of 17, she was seriously wounded by being accidentally shot by a friend goofing around with a gun. This was a life-changing experience for her. She will never forget the nurses who took care of her during that very difficult time. She has been a registered nurse since 1989. She has worked in high-risk Labor and Delivery, as well as maternal home health, including home phototherapy for newborns. She recently obtained her International Board of Certified Lactation Consultants certificate, and has opened up a postpartum breastfeeding clinic at her hospital serving the local community. This job is her passion. She has been married to her husband for 20 years and they have two wonderful children.

HEATHER TEMPEST, RN, PNC(C), has been an obstetrical nurse for nearly 30 years, specializing primarily in Labor and Delivery. She completed her nursing training in 1979 at Ryerson Polytechnical Institute and received a specialty certificate in Maternal Newborn Care, as well as a diploma in Healthcare Administration from the Ontario Hospital Association. Heather is active on many committees, advocating for optimum care of mothers and their newborns. She is an active participant in perinatal bereavement care, assisting families through their difficult loss. Heather lives in Toronto, Ontario, and has two grown children.

Labor of Love

A Midwife's Memoir

~

Cara Muhlhahn

Foreword by Abby Epstein and Ricki Lake

Chapter 9

~

A Day in the Life

Here's what a typical home visit is like. Marina, a patient who lives in Howard Beach, Queens, is in her first trimester with her fifth child. Marina has been looking forward to our visit. It is not our first time working together; I've already delivered three of her four kids, and I'm about to deliver another one for her. It is easy to park here. I just pull right up in front of the house, although here the neighbors definitely watch carefully. They want to make sure I meet with their approval.

I knock on the door of her basement apartment. When I enter, Marina is teaching the kids at the kitchen table. She homeschools them. I get to see all the girls. How they have grown since the last time I've seen them—it's been over a year, maybe even two! But I saw Marina more recently, as she had assisted at the birth of a woman from her church. I love seeing her, and she is just as happy to see me.

Marina loves being pregnant, and I enjoy her glow. Before we officially start the prenatal visit, though, her daughters treat me to a little show-and-tell. There's a princess costume, a book, and a review of the play they put on last week. I am their special guest. The girls scramble for the floor to give all of the important news to me. I sit on the floor with them. I'm not really a chair person. I have to greet the cat, too, although he's definitely not taking to my presence as well as the girls are.

We planned this particular visit for a time when Valnn, Marina's husband, could be present. He is a public school teacher and talks proudly about informing his middle school science students of his wife's pregnancy and their plans for a homebirth. It's like a big reunion. Aurora, their oldest daughter, and Liam are the same age. Aurora is starting to bloom. Marina tells me she behaves like Hitler with lipstick. We commiserate kindly about the challenges of raising a tween.

After I take out her chart—I don't need to repeat her history because I have it all down on paper from her previous pregnancies—we go straight to calculating the due date. We drag out the calendars to be sure about the first day of her last menstrual period. The last thing we want is any lack of certainty that might make it appear, down the line, as if Marina is overdue when she's not. We go over their schedules closely. Was Valnn away at any point, and if so, when did he return? We figure after four kids together, this one is not the milkman's. We can joke like that because we have a mutual trust. And the trust between a midwife and her expectant family is given and taken seriously and with honor.

After we catch up on whatever details I need to know to estimate the due date accurately, the black "doctor bag" comes out. All the kids know it. They have all had the chance to dig into it and remove the tools: a fetoscope, a stethoscope, a blood pressure cuff, and a measuring tape. The toddlers drag these things around while I have Marina lie down on the couch. Since she is under 20 weeks, we don't need to use my measuring tape, which is housed in a whimsical plastic pig. Pull it out by its curlicue tail; roll it back up by pressing on its nose. I like using fun tools because they appeal to kids who are about to have new siblings.

When it's time to listen to the heartbeat, we try with the fetoscope. Even though books and teachers will say that the fetal heartbeat can't be heard with the fetoscope before 20 weeks, I have heard it as early as 15. Marina would prefer not to expose the baby to an unnecessary ultrasound.

We can hear it! It is very faint, so we turn down the radio, and the kids have to stay very, very still, waiting their turn to listen. It's thrilling to witness their excitement. Some of them hear it; some do not. Marina and Valnn do. It's interesting: Even with all of the proof—a missed period, a positive pregnancy test, nausea, fatigue—so many women remain uncertain that the pregnancy is a reality until the first time they hear the heartbeat.

If we couldn't hear the heartbeat with the fetoscope, we might have heard it on the Doppler, which I bring to each visit in case. The Doppler is a handheld six-inch sonar device with a wand that can be placed on the abdomen and used for monitoring. Marina's blood pressure is normal, as it has been with each pregnancy. I write down my data. We look at our calendars to consider times for our next visit, and discuss what, if anything, she may need to prepare for.

I have been at Marina's about an hour. I explain to the kids that I will be coming back soon. As I drive away, I wave good-bye to one of the girls, Maya, from the window of her grandma's apartment upstairs. I had to wait for her to install herself in the window before driving away. We wave furiously and all is well. I've got about 30 minutes to get to my next appointment.

THAT'S USUALLY HOW IT GOES: 45 minutes to an hour with each patient and 30 minutes travel time in between. It allows me to see four to six patients a day, which is very manageable. It also allows me to spend quality time with them in the comfort of their own environments. Of course, that's a much lower census than in most busy doctor's offices. They may see 20 or more patients in a day for mere minutes each. The patients usually have to wait a half hour or so for the doctor to come in while they're cold, dressed in nothing but a hospital gown, and seated uncomfortably on a table.

I'm not getting rich doing this. I certainly don't bring in doctor's wages. But that was never the point. Offering women honesty, choices, comfort, and personalized, high-quality care satisfies my soul in a way being a doctor never would have.

The satisfaction I get from midwifery makes it worth the high degree of dedication and sacrifice. My work takes a lot out of me. But I like the adventure that midwifery brings to my life. I like having to drop everything to answer to a higher calling, the ruggedness of hard work, and the idea that when nature calls, there is no choice but to answer.

Don't get me wrong—I'm not always found in a perfect state of grace when the pager goes off and I have to jump. Sometimes, it's hard to rally, like when a primip calls when she is in what I know are the very early stages of labor. I don't always want to get in the car and go all the way to the Bronx to see her, spend three hours with her, and then go home because she's only one centimeter dilated. I know I'm going to lose my parking space and maybe not find one where she is. In those moments, I call on something I learned from my mother: *Do the action and the feeling will follow.* When I lack the willingness to do a particular good deed, I just do the deed, and the feeling comes afterward. It's one of the few Catholic-school lessons my mother truly valued, and it works. Once I'm in the car and on my way there, it hits me: this first-time mom, who has no idea what to expect, is going to feel so much better with me there to suss out her situation and tell her what to expect next. My crankiness melts away.

It's hard to describe the satisfaction I get from my work in a way that does it justice. I find it absolutely thrilling both to facilitate and witness the triumph a mother experiences when she delivers her child naturally in the support and comfort of her home environment. Those feelings are what make me okay with doing crazy things like spending whole days killing time in people's neighborhoods or sleeping in my car overnight, around the corner from them, so that I'll be near enough to a patient when she is ready to deliver. I've slept in my car several times after I've had an evening phone conversation with a mom in labor, usually a multip, because things often turn the corner very quickly from the beginning of active labor to delivery. Rather than put pressure on her to know when to call next, I head her way a little early so that I don't have to feel rushed if she calls me and things are going quickly.

I can't sleep in my bed at home knowing that I might be needed, so sleeping in the car reduces my anxiety and allows me to rest at least a little. There have been times when my radar was off, and I slept in the car only to go right back home in the morning. I then had to come back the following day for the birth. I never let the parents know that I am doing this because I am trying to avoid the fishbowl effect.

If I were to go to a woman in labor's home and nothing was happening, I might actually get in the way. Many women, with their midwife on hand, would feel pressured to make something happen and guilty for calling too early. By getting in my car ahead of the game and hanging out there until the next call, I'm taking the pressure off the mom, while also making sure I don't miss the birth if she figures out very late in the game that it's time to call the midwife. Sometimes people look completely shocked at the speed of my transit time, but they are always grateful.

These overnights have given birth to a little fantasy about going on *Pimp My Ride*, the MTV reality show where they customize cars in cool ways. I would ask for a backseat that pulls out partway into a really comfortable bed. There would need to be some kind of electrically controlled shade system and a refrigerator that runs off the car battery to keep things cold throughout the night. A satellite traffic alert system would be great, as would a heating system that doesn't cause emissions. And, of course, a sign that lets me park wherever I need to, whenever I need to. And I'll take a siren, too, thank you very much.

I REMEMBER SLEEPING in my car one time in Queens around Christmastime. A mom there was having her second baby. She called and said she was just beginning to have contractions. They were regular but still only seven minutes apart. She said she'd call if there was any change.

Looking at my clock, I figured that change she was waiting for might come right around morning rush hour, and I didn't want to feel anxious about driving on the Long Island Expressway in that kind of traffic. So I went to her neighborhood, parked, and slept in the car.

By 10 the next morning, to my surprise, I hadn't heard from her. I called and asked if I could just come and check on her. She said things had slowed down, but she okayed my visit. When I got there, the tree was up, and her sister-in-law, who'd had a homebirth many years ago, was there. After I arrived, I noticed that the mom would wander into the other room quietly about every five minutes. It's not unusual for laboring moms to need to get away from everyone. But I started to get suspicious that something more was going on, and I asked if I could check her. She was fully dilated and had the baby about 30 minutes later. It turned out the only reason she didn't have an urge to push was because her water hadn't broken. When it finally did, things happened *fast*.

Because she was a multip, I could very easily have missed that birth if I hadn't been just around the corner. It's such an easy—and unfortunate—mistake to make. The mom says everything's okay, because it is. But if that water breaks, the baby is out in three minutes. Times like that, I ask that the woman lie down while I'm in transit to try to slow things down.

Beth, a woman having her third baby, lived on the Upper West Side. Getting from the Lower East Side, where I am, to the Upper West Side is one of the worst commutes in all of Manhattan. Beth called me at 9 PM and said that she didn't need me yet, although she had been contracting mildly all day. There was bloody show. She just wanted to give me a heads-up. I quickly got in the car and on my way. I was with Jenna, a dear friend, an East Village compatriot, and my favorite doula, whom Beth had hired. As we were crossing Central Park, Beth paged me. Since I was driving, Jenna called her right back. I listened carefully to Jenna's side of the conversation, gauging the action by her responses. Beth said something, and Jenna inferred that Beth's water had broken.

In her reassuring way, Jenna said, "That's good."

Then I said out loud, "No it's not!" Pedal to the metal, we made it to Beth's 11 minutes before the birth.

Another time, I parked myself for the day on Staten Island for a mom whose last birth I'd missed by three minutes—one of only two births I have ever missed. She called in the morning to say her water had broken, and I jumped in the car. I wasn't going to miss this one, too. I went to her home to check on the baby. After I had evaluated the baby as stable and set up a system for relaying information about baby movement and temperatures, instead of going back to my home office, I went to a nearby park to read. I decided to kill the day on Staten Island.

We spoke several times on the phone, but nothing was happening. My patient had no idea where I was when we spoke. She went for a walk in the park with her family. Still, nothing. Until about 4 o'clock in the afternoon.

The mom went back home to relax, and her husband took their three daughters to the Shaolin Temple for their regular lessons. Her mother, visiting from Italy for the special event, went up to nap on the third floor of their home. With no one around, my patient went into labor. She had the baby about 30 minutes after she called me with contractions. I was glad I was close enough to get there in time.

Not all homebirth moms are multips with quick second, third—or seventh—labors. Many times, I spend at least 24 hours at a family's house while a primip is in labor. I might need to monitor a mom or a baby particularly closely. In those situations, I need to be on-site. Depending upon how well I know the family, there's the potential for awkward moments. Sometimes I just need to crash and get a couple of hours of shut-eye, or I'm just starving and need to eat whatever they've got in the fridge.

Sometimes, when I say, "Okay, I'm going to take a nap," and get ready to lie down somewhere in their apartment, I'll get a concerned look from the dad or the grandmother. But it's what I've got to do. I've learned not to be bashful about that. I am able to stay awake for long periods of time and still function, but I've also developed discipline. I know I have to take care of my needs so that I'm able to be at the top of my game when the crucial moments roll around.

I try to get the other people who are there in support of the mother to take care of themselves, too. People watching a birth have a natural tendency to feel guilty about resting or eating when the person they love is going through labor. They're so conflicted, because they feel as if they have to be completely selfless and suffer along with her. But I tell them that to help her, they need to maintain their own energy levels. They often seem relieved to be given permission for things as basic as sleeping and eating.

WHEN I'M OUT AT A patient's apartment for hours and hours, or overnight, I'm not the only one sacrificing. My kid is, too. His whole life, Liam has had to deal with having a single mom who's on call 24/7. Since I began, though, I have always known the importance of making time for Liam.

The year I opened my practice, I asked Miriam if she could cover for me during August, just for patients' questions or emergency visits. I don't schedule appointments or take patients who will deliver in August. For the past two years, I've added February as a second month off.

Miriam said, "Cara, you can't take a month off in your first year of practice!"

"Watch me!" I replied. I yearned for the downtime of motherhood: cooking, reading, swimming, and just hanging out with my kid. And, I needed to decompress from the demands of pager-dominated living. In recent years, Liam and I have spent my two months off together in Costa Rica. It helps to be too far away to be called into action. During my time in New York, there are no weekends away or off , just the ritual of Sunday night salsa dancing to my favorite Afro-Cuban band Nu Guajiro. And even then, I'm still on call, so I have to be careful with the libations.

Liam deserves a medal. Granted, his father is also very much involved in raising him and often covers for me when I'm not around. And for Liam's first five years, I always had an au pair living with us, which made it easier to handle overnight deliveries and other situations in which I wasn't available for him. But I know it has been hard for Liam. He has always known that that beeper can go off at any time, and then he has to be second priority.

Liam's a real trouper, though, and he has been from an early age. I think I might have passed down to him the soul of a person in service, something I believe I inherited from my mother, who taught young men in prison for many years after my parents divorced.

There was one particular experience when Liam was three that inspires me so much. I got paged late at night, and I said, "Honey, I'm gonna have to go help a mom push a baby out." This is how I always said it because I often feel it's disempowering to a mother for me to say that I'm delivering her baby. No, she is.

Liam looked at me with these sad, puppy-dog eyes and said, "Oh, Mom, don't go!" But before I could even respond, he changed his expression and said, "No—you have to go."

I think he takes pride vicariously in what I do. He knows that I'm providing a service. And he knows that he's part of it because I constantly acknowledge that he makes sacrifices for me.

But it hasn't always been so easy for him to adjust, like when I haven't been there when he woke up, or for dinner, or for Christmas. When he was about four, I did miss Christmas. A woman in Larchmont, up in Westchester County, was having her second baby. She broke her water on December 23, which was before her due date. She went into labor before I had a chance to culture her for beta strep, a potentially lethal bacteria that up to 30 percent of women can carry. I had seen her a few days before, during a blizzard, when I didn't have my prenatal bag because I'd just come from a labor. I figured I'd come back the following week to culture her, but her water broke before I had a chance to return.

Now I had a bit of a clinical challenge on my hands. I had to watch her carefully to make sure the baby wasn't at risk and to put her lawyer husband at ease. So the day before Christmas, there I was, heading to Larchmont. The mother didn't go into labor right away, even though it was her second baby. I gave her castor oil, and still nothing. In the meantime, I was giving her an antibiotic every four to six hours just as a precaution so that if she did have beta strep, the baby wouldn't get it.

At a certain point, I realized I wasn't going to make it home for Christmas. I hadn't even gotten Liam any presents, not to mention a tree. In my family, we had always maintained a tradition of getting a Christmas tree at the very last minute because we could get a bargain. It's a tradition I've kept up as an homage to my father.

I called Geoff and said, "Why don't you take Liam to your mom's house for Christmas?" They always had a nice Christmas celebration. He agreed, and they spent the day at Geoff's parents'.

Late on Christmas Day, the baby was born. I finally made it home on the twenty-sixth. Liam and Geoff met me at the apartment. As soon as I got to the door, Liam asked me, so innocently, "Mom, why didn't Santy Claus come?"

My eyes welled with tears and my throat constricted, but I held it together. "Well," I told him, "because I was at a birth, and so all the doors were locked and he couldn't get in."

He thought a second, and then asked, "But, Mom, don't we have a chim-uh-ney?" My heart was broken. I didn't know what more to say. At a later date, Nicole, the birth mom, wrote him a beautiful letter expressing her gratitude for Liam having been without his mom on Christmas Day.

Because of my demanding work, Liam has had many surrogate parents and families in his young life. While away from him, I have always loved and missed him deeply. I arranged my professional life in such a way as to be able to spend as much time with Liam as I could. I did prenatal visits when he was in school so that I would be done with work by the time he needed to be picked up.

I always tried to create as normal a home life as possible, helping him with his homework, having dinner with him, watching his favorite shows with him. But the pager has always kept things unpredictable, so I've needed a whole backup network of babysitters.

When Liam was in pre-K, I attended a kid's birthday party where I met many moms, among them my now dear friend Elida, a soulful woman with a great heart. She was a stay-at-home mom who lived on my block, and she has a beautiful daughter who was in the same school Liam attended, The Neighborhood School. We clicked, and I proposed the job of babysitter/backup mom to her. We made a mutually acceptable financial arrangement and worked together for quite a few years while Liam was in elementary school.

If I had a labor while Liam was in school, I would call Elida. She would pick him up and take him home to her house after school. In the middle of the night, I would call and wake her, apologetically. I'd drive Liam down half a block, often handing him to her wrapped in a down comforter, and run back to my car, always in a hurry.

One time, in my haste to get to a laboring mother, I fell on my butt on the stairs with Liam in my arms. He hit his leg, and it got scratched. Poor guy.

In his half stupor, he cried out, "Why did you do that, Mom?"

And all I could say was, "It was a mistake. This is an emergency and I was moving too fast, and that's it. I can't be a nice mommy right now." I felt terrible, but I knew I just had to get out of there right then.

Liam remembers that, and I think he mostly derives pride from it. A few years later, I was walking him and his friend Luca home from school. It was just days after I had done my first neonatal resuscitation at home, and I had told Liam about it. On the walk home, a few steps ahead of the boys, I heard Liam tell his friend very proudly, "My mom saves lives."

WHEN ELIDA TIRED OF being on call for me, which anyone would have sooner or later, Carol, another fellow single mom friend, took over. She lived only about two blocks away, and Liam was friends with her son, Lateef, whom I had delivered. With the new arrangement, the kids got to enjoy occasional sleepovers and walks to school together.

I will always feel indebted to all of the people who have helped me out in this way. Even though they were all paid fairly, I know that they watched Liam and rolled with the punches of my unpredictable schedule out of the goodness of their hearts.

IT'S NOT JUST LIAM I'VE LOST precious moments with. I missed my grandmother's passing. I recently received a letter of appreciation from the mother who was in labor that day. She hadn't known that my grandma was dying as her son was being born, and why should she have? I had kept it to myself.

She was a primip, and it was a long labor. We were both tired, and so we laid down—she on the bed, breathing through her contractions, and I, on the floor, wondering how my family felt about my not showing up for my grandmother's last moments. But Nanager lived in Ohio. There was no way I could leave to be by her side while on call. Yes, I suppose I could have asked Miriam to cover me, but it's not that easy to leave a woman in her time of need.

I also nearly missed my mother's passing. It was in March of 1997, when I was 40 and my practice was young. My mother had lung cancer and was very sick. She had decided to die at home, which seems fitting to me in so many ways. I wanted to go visit her, and I made a couple of attempts. I told the two patients who were ready to go about my trip, reassuring them that I would be able to make it back from Ithaca—which is about three and a half hours from the city—in no time. I told Miriam I was going, so that if anything happened and I couldn't make it, she would be ready. But pregnant women are skittish.

The first time I attempted to make the journey, one of the two patients, who was having her seventh baby, paged me reporting the kind of contractions that could inconclusively indicate false labor or early labor. So an hour and a half north of New York City, I turned around, only to realize when I got to her house that it was just her nerves playing with her. The next time I went to see my mother, I made it all the way to Ithaca. But then, in the middle of the night, one of my patients paged me with contractions.

So I drove back maniacally in about three hours—and, of course, she never went into labor, either.

By the time I did get to my mom's bedside, she was already in a coma. I had missed her last days of consciousness. I don't know if I've forgiven myself for this.

I wailed at my mother's bedside. I spoke to her because I learned in nursing school that hearing is the last sense to go. I was trying to think of what to say or do to soothe her, when I remembered that when we were kids, she used to sing "Danny Boy" to us to put us to sleep at night. So after telling her that it was okay to let go, that she had been a good person in her life, and she shouldn't be afraid, I began singing. She then exhaled for the last time. And strangely, on cue, "Danny Boy" began playing on the radio upstairs. I got chills. I hadn't even realized that it was Saint Patrick's Day. It was a very eerie yet lovely way to say goodbye.

Share Your Stories
with Kaplan Publishing

KAPLAN PUBLISHING, THE #1 educational resource for nurses, would like to feature your story in an upcoming anthology in the *Kaplan Voices: Nurses* series. Please share the stories behind the relationships, experiences, and issues you encounter on the job — whether you work in a hospital, clinic, home setting, hospice, private medical practice, or elsewhere.

Entertaining and educational, inspirational and practical, each *Kaplan Voices: Nurses* anthology features true stories written by nurses about the experiences and relationships that inspire and enrich their lives and all those who come into contact with them.

FOR WRITER'S GUIDELINES or to join our mailing list, please contact Kaplan Publishing by email at *kaplanvoicesnurses@gmail.com*, or write to us at:

Nurse Stories
Editorial Assistant
Kaplan Publishing
1 Liberty Plaza, 24th Floor
New York, NY 10006, USA